ADULT
OBESITY
THERAPY

Pergamon Titles of Related Interest

Agras EATING DISORDERS:
Management of Obesity, Bulimia and Anorexia Nervosa

Kirschenbaum/Johnson/Stalonas TREATING CHILDHOOD AND
ADOLESCENT OBESITY

Weiss/Katzman/Wolchik TREATING BULIMIA:
A Psychoeducational Approach

Related Journal
(Free sample copies available upon request)

CLINICAL PSYCHOLOGY REVIEW

PSYCHOLOGY PRACTITIONER GUIDEBOOKS

EDITORS

Arnold P. Goldstein, Syracuse University
Leonard Krasner, Stanford University & SUNY at Stony Brook
Sol L. Garfield, Washington University in St. Louis

ADULT OBESITY THERAPY

MICHAEL D. LEBOW
University of Manitoba

PERGAMON PRESS
New York • Oxford • Beijing • Frankfurt
São Paulo • Sydney • Tokyo • Toronto

Pergamon Press Offices:

U.S.A.	Pergamon Press, Inc., Maxwell House, Fairview Park, Elmsford, New York 10523, U.S.A.
U.K.	Pergamon Press plc, Headington Hill Hall, Oxford OX3 0BW, England
PEOPLE'S REPUBLIC OF CHINA	Pergamon Press, Qianmen Hotel, Beijing, People's Republic of China
FEDERAL REPUBLIC OF GERMANY	Pergamon Press GmbH, Hammerweg 6, D-6242 Kronberg, Federal Republic of Germany
BRAZIL	Pergamon Editora Ltda, Rua Eça de Queiros, 346, CEP 04011, São Paulo, Brazil
AUSTRALIA	Pergamon Press Australia Pty Ltd., P.O. Box 544, Potts Point, NSW 2011, Australia
JAPAN	Pergamon Press, 8th Floor, Matsuoka Central Building, 1-7-1 Nishishinjuku, Shinjuku-ku, Tokyo 160, Japan
CANADA	Pergamon Press Canada Ltd., Suite 271, 253 College Street, Toronto, Ontario M5T 1R5, Canada

Library of Congress Cataloging in Publication Data

LeBow, Michael D.
    Adult obesity therapy / Michael D. LeBow.
      p. cm. -- (Psychology practitioners guidebooks)
    Includes index.
    ISBN 0-08-035556-0 : ISBN 0-08-035555-2 (pbk.)
    1. Obesity--Treatment. 2. Psychotherapy. 3. Behavior therapy.
4. Reducing. I. Title. II. Series.
    [DNLM: 1. Behavior Therapy--in adulthood. 2. Obesity--in
adulthood. WD 210 L449a]
RC552.025L39 1989
616.3'9806--dc19
DNLM/DLC
for Library of Congress
                                          88-22423
                                            CIP

Printed in the United States of America

Dedication

To Mom and Dad Ernest

Contents

Preface

Numbers of individuals desperately want to reduce. To do so, many consult a health care professional for assistance, some while they are already in therapy for other problems and some anew just for weight loss itself. In either circumstance, practitioners cannot offer universally effective remedies for obesity. Indeed, the history of this treatment is spotty: successes, partial successes, and failures coexist.

What such treatment can offer, however, is support as well as safe and useful practices with potential to change body shape. Especially when given in tailored combinations, these strategies may be of help to many. To maximize the possibility of salutary outcomes, therapists must fit available resources to the needs of their clients. One attempt to do so is the subject of this guidebook.

After an introduction to obesity and an exposition of tactics frequently used in attempting to treat it, the book addresses the tailoring issue. As regards this, the next five chapters discuss drawing the client into the therapy process and also analyze, in turn, body, energy, and behavioral variables. Typical client–therapist dialogue and discussion, along with illustrative commentary, buttress these examinations. The final chapter tackles the perplexing issue of follow-through. Finally, the reader will find eight appendices that are of service in delivering the various facets of weight-control therapy.

I want this book to be welcomed by health care professionals as a conservative, practical guide for helping their overweight clients. The approach put forward is no panacea but is a logical extension of many currently available methods. Although it has been the mainstay of the Manitoba Obesity Clinic for years, it has not yet been critically evaluated. I hope this narrative stimulates this evaluation. Needed are better procedures of treatment, continuance, and maintenance so that therapists are able to move ahead in offering their obese clients effective solutions.

This book would be impossible to write were it not for the many researchers and practitioners who have labored to improve the quality of obesity care. I am indebted to them.

I am also indebted to the numerous graduate students who have worked with me over the years to make the Manitoba Obesity Clinic a reasonable alternative for the overweight in this community.

Lastly, I want to say to my two special friends David and Ray and to my family Barbara, Bill and Matt, thank you for supporting my struggle to overcome pain. Thank you for easing my burden. Thank you for caring.

Michael D. LeBow
Winnipeg 1988

One

The Obesity Situation

There are legions of overweight adults in the United States alone—approximately 34 million (NIH, 1985), more than the entire population of some industrialized countries (e.g., Canada). Similarly, using the prevalence data of the National Health and Nutrition surveys of 1971–1974 and 1976–1980 (NHANES I & II), Simopoulos puts the figure for overweight adults in this country at 32.6 million. She points out that 11.5 million are "severely overweight." Recent estimates are that one out of five in the United States is overweight (Agras, 1987) and that approximately a third of American adults need to be treated for obesity (Jeffery, 1987 assessing NIH 1985 findings).

SOCIETAL CONNECTIONS

Data on the incidence of obesity are complexly related to such variables as sex, age, class, income, education, and race. For instance, prevalence has been linked with affluence. Scrutinizing results from the Midtown Manhattan Study (Srole, Langer, Michael, Opler, & Rennie, 1962), Stunkard and colleagues (Goldblatt, Moore, & Stunkard, 1965; Moore, Stunkard, & Srole, 1962) have led the way in showing a relationship between social class and obesity. The association they have described is strongest for the adult woman. Measuring weight for height, Stunkard and colleagues disclosed that the overweight compared with their lighter peers had a lower socioeconomic status (income, occupation, rent). Likewise, using the Techumseh Community Health Survey as well as data from the Ten-State Nutrition Study on thousands of individuals and measuring fatness per se, Garn (1985) indicated that fatter women were in low-income groups. They were much fatter than wealthier women. During adolescence (see also Garn & Clark, 1975; Garn, Hopkins, & Ryan, 1981) the poorer girls appeared to be fatter and seemed to remain fatter when they reached adulthood, particularly if they stayed poor.

1

Even if these poorer young females were thin in their early years, they tended to become fatter if they stayed poor. For the richer females, the outcome is different. As adults they were thin, no matter if they were fat as adolescents—a finding Garn refers to as an "income related reversal of relative fatness."

Whereas Garn (1985) finds a negative relationship between income (as well as education) and fatness for women, he describes a positive one for adult men (but see Forman, Trowbridge, Gentry, Marks, & Hogelin, 1986). Van Itallie's (1985) disclosures, based on NHANES data, are in line with those of Garn. Van Itallie also looked at racial variables, noting that the incidence of overweight was higher among black women compared with white women—regardless at which age testing occurred. For men, something like the result for women, albeit less marked, appeared, except that for the men there was an age effect: racial differences inter-twined with the prevalence of overweight for the 35- to 55-year-olds.

Garn further showed that for women, economic level and race inde-pendently predicted overweight. Also looking at race and sex and evaluating the behavioral risk factor survey data, Forman et al. (1986) found that for Whites in the 18–49 age group, greater numbers of males compared with females were overweight. The opposite occurred if the comparison was for Blacks and Hispanics. Within these cohorts, more females were overweight, except for those in the 30- to 39-year-old range.

That the foregoing variables and obesity are connected is indisput-able. But it is also clear that they are intricately connected, and that studies about the connections disagree. Differences in the data obtained reflect, in part, differences among researchers in defining and measuring obesity and in assessing many of the variables to which they believe it is linked. Nonetheless, there is little doubt that overweight and obesity are, no pun intended, immense problems. And there are data on young-sters and teenagers, as well as adults, showing it to be increasing (Dietz, Gortmaker, Sobol, & Wehler, 1985; Simopoulos, 1986).

OBESITY: PHYSIOLOGICAL ROOTS

When an individual's "whole adipose tissue mass (adipose organ) is enlarged out of proportion to other body tissues" (Lloyd & Wolff, 1980), he or she is obese. Put simply, obesity is excessive fatness. Body fat is stored as triglyceride in fat cells (adipocytes). When mobilized, fat pro-vides the bearer with energy, over 90% (Bray, 1985), energy to fuel meta-bolic functions and voluntary pursuits.

Of Fat Cells

Despite criticism of methods (Gurr & Kirtland, 1978; Roche, 1981) as well as contradictory data and opinion (Ashwell, Priest, & Bondoux, 1975; Garn, Clark, & Guire, 1975), we can state that fat individuals can be described by the anatomy of their adipose tissue. The hypertrophically obese have excessively large fat cells. For them, surplus calories have culminated in the enlargement of adipose tissue through triglyceride storage in already existing fat cells—hypertrophy. The surplus can also help trigger the formation of new fat cells—hyperplasia. Persons so affected are hyperplastically obese. Many fat adults who became fat as adults evidence fat cell hypertrophy, whereas many fat adults who became fat as children show fat cell hyperplasia (Salans, Cushman, & Weismann, 1973). Some individuals are both hypertrophically and hyperplastically obese (see Brownell, 1982; Knittle, 1975; Powers, 1980).

Critical periods for the multiplication of fat cells have been proposed, including the third trimester, childhood, and adolescence. An increase in fat cell number may also, as Sjostrom (1980) in his review seems to suggest, take place during adulthood. Indeed, that there are persons possessing exaggerated numbers of fat cells who became obese as adults marks the inexactitude of the relationship between age of obesity onset and fat-cell hyperplasia (Hirsch, 1975).

What's of most concern is the finding that weight loss is associated with a shrinkage, not diminution, of fat cells. In fact, weight losses may cease when fat cells are shrunk to normal sizes, leaving obese many of the already hyperplastically obese (Bjorntorp, Carlgren, Isaksson, Krotiewski, Larsson, & Sjostrom, 1975). Adipocyte numbers do not appear to decrease. That may mean that in order to stay thin, the hyperplastically obese adult would have to unduly restrict food intake. Doing so in our food-laden environment would be most difficult.

Difficult at least because, as Jordan (1973) and Nisbett (1972, 1974) articulate, the body resists any voluntary attempts to maintain disequilibrium. It seeks to restore the disequilibrium caused by long-term calorie restriction, perhaps through a decreasing energy expenditure rate (Keesey, 1980).

Of Setpoints

In other words, words that still mean resisting change, one may say that the body appears to muster a metabolic defense against weight loss—its *setpoint* (see Keesey & Corbett, 1984). The term setpoint, from systems engineering, is a theoretical construct. It is used to describe the apparent stability of a person's weight over time (Keesey, 1980) and, relatedly, the great difficulty of trying to maintain an alteration of it, be it upward or downward. The setpoint for body weight is thought to be the weight below which the body tends to gain and above which it tends to lose; the analogy is to a thermostat and where on it the point is set.

Setpoint theory says that there are internal pressures upon individuals who have managed to change or are in the throes of changing their weights. These pressures are to return to previous levels, to body weight setpoints—lower weights for the gainers, higher weights for the reducers. For example, Sims and Horton (1968) studied the problems their subjects, prison volunteers, had gaining weight. The men were fed large amounts of food, much more than is customary in jail. Significantly higher weights could not be maintained or, in some of the men, even reached. The simple, calorie-based arithmetic of weight gain failed to predict the body changes that resulted.

Looking at the opposite circumstance, the one of most interest to obesity therapists, Keys, Brozek, Henschel, Mickelson, and Taylor (1950) showed, in their classic account, that the body resists long-term changes in weight. The authors subjected their male participants to a period of semistarvation lasting months. Although weights initially decreased, they eventually stabilized, even though calorie intakes remained low. Significantly, basal metabolic rates (for each subject, this is the energy output of the body at rest after a 12-hour fast) decreased beyond what would be expected from simply losing size (see Keesey, 1980). The body, it seems, adjusted to the lowered energy intake by lowering rate of energy expenditure—a defensive response.

WHO ARE THE OBESE AND OVERWEIGHT?

Techniques for picking out the obese range from simple to complex; some are highly intrusive (see Bray, 1976, 1985; Forbes, 1962; Garrow, 1974, 1978a; Powers, 1980). The easiest way is estimating by visual inspection. The obese person or someone else doing the examination looks for enlarged sites of fat deposition. Yet estimating by inspecting disallows quantification—that is, discovering what percentage of one's weight is fat.

The most direct and precise way to analyze body constituents—to describe how much fat tissue someone has—is autopsy. But for each candidate, this obviously is a one-time affair precluding pre–post treatment evaluations. Volunteers are few.

Less macabre and more conducive to repeated measurements are the indirect methods for studying body fat—among these are isotope and chemical dilution techniques, which use fat-soluble gases (cyclopropane), and the densitometric procedure. Densitometry, Behnke's method, requires weighing the subject in and out of water—fat in contrast to other tissues is lighter than water—and correcting for residual air in the lungs and intestine (Goldman & Buskirk, 1959). Although these indirect assessment tactics may disagree on how fat the same person is, they are currently among the most precise of the laboratory practices available.

Anthropometric Assessments

There are several ways anthropometric measures are made, including determining circumferences of the waist, chest (bust), arms, hips, and thighs (see box 4.2) and the thicknesses of skinfolds. The latter, skinfold calipering, is relatively simple to do (see chapter 4 for sites and suggestions). The practice of assessing skinfolds rests upon the degree of the relationship presumed between subcutaneous and total body fat.

To use the results of one or other of the more complex fat estimation methods (e.g., densitometry) as the criterion to which to correlate skinfold results, some combined with other anthropometric data, researchers apply a prediction formula. This formula is based upon the weighted combinations of the specific skinfolds taken and the other anthropometric indices (e.g., Zuti & Golding, 1973). The accuracy of predicting fatness in this way varies (Brozek & Keys, 1951; Moody, Kollias, & Buskirk, 1968). Nonetheless, tabulating skinfolds helps researchers and therapists track the changes in the body wrought by treatment.

Weight and Height Indices

Another class of anthropometric measurements, the most extensively used class (Bray, 1985), is weight to height and its correlation with body fat. Weight–height indices are often part of the data sets of large epidemiologic studies, ones examining the deleterious effects of overweight and obesity on physical health. Overweight is weight in excess of some standard based upon height, age, sex, and frame-size. The source of standards is often the 1959 or 1983 Metropolitan Life Insurance tables of desirable weight.

Overweight is different from overfat. In our programs of treatment, clients are taught that a person may be overweight to some degree without being overfat to any great degree. A well-muscled man, for instance, may be heavy for height but in no way too fat; conversely, someone may be overfat and not too heavy at all (e.g., an inactive person). Heaviness and corpulence are therefore distinguished. Clients learn that the scale reflects both their fat and lean tissue weights. Two individuals, the same or different ages but equal in weight, may well differ in clothing sizes because of the amounts of lean and adipose tissue their total body weights reflect. Taking heaviness for fatness is, as clients find out, sometimes an error. Although, they also learn, when someone is very obese, he or she is undoubtedly overweight, too (Van Itallie, 1985).

At the upper ranges of weight distribution, overweight and overfat likely coexist. An agreed upon benchmark is 20% overweight,[1] though some professionals opt for a greater percentage of excess. Weight for height has often been used by investigators as *the* descriptor of obesity (see below) as well as *the* metric for determining mortality ratios and health risks. Clearly, weight tables are of value in determining obesity and the need for treatment (NIH, 1985).

Relative Weight and Body Mass

Of the derived indices based upon weight in relation to height that correlate well with body fat (Bray, 1985), *relative weight*—Metropolitan relative weight (Simopoulos, 1986)—and *body mass* are favorites to compute. Relative weight is the ratio of actual to desirable weight converted to a percent figure. Desirable weight is the weight associated with minimum mortality for an individual of a particular height and sex. Desirable weight is often set as the midpoint of the middle frame-size category of the Metropolitan Life desirable weight tables. One problem with the tables is that, being based on only policyholders, they do not necessarily mirror the mortality experience of adult Americans in general (NIH, 1985).

Most preferable of the weight-based estimates of obesity is Quetelet's body mass index (BMI).

$$\text{Body mass} = \frac{\text{weight in kilograms}}{\text{height in meters}^2}$$

Its high correlation with body fat and low correlation with height make it quite useful (NIH, 1985; Simopoulos, 1986).

Bray (1985) says overweight is having a BMI of 25–30 and obesity is falling above a BMI range of 30. Simopoulos (1986), using NHANES data on a reference group of 20–29 year olds, likens overweight in men to

---

[1]When I use the term obesity I mean excessively fat and/or overweight by at least 20%. Particularly in later chapters of this narrative, I use overweight and obesity synonymously for style, recognizing that their precise definitions differ. By far, most of the clients I see— the sources of most of the information presented in later chapters—are 20% or more overweight.

possessing a BMI at or higher than 28 and in women to a BMI of 34. The data from which the BMI for women is computed uses the power function of 1.5. Severe overweight in women, employing this lower power function, is, for Simopoulos, a BMI of 42 or greater; in men, using the more customary exponent of two, it is 32. As does Simopoulos, Van Itallie (1985), reporting NHANES data, defines overweight and severe overweight in BMI terms. Applying the meters squared formula, he indicates that the data show cutoff points for women of 27.3 (overweight) and 32.3 (severely overweight). Uniform definitions of obesity based on BMI are therefore unavailable, a situation inhibiting comparisons among studies as well as advances in obesity research (Jamieson, 1987).

Using the 1983 Metropolitan tables, the tables reproduced in appendix 1, the BMI corresponding to the benchmark of 20% above desirable weight is—applying the power function of two—27.2 for men and 26.9 for women (NIH, 1985). For Agras (1987), who reports a translation of the Metropolitan height and weight tables into BMI percentiles, men falling within the BMI range of 26–28 are potential treatment candidates; the range is 25–28 for women.

As BMIs exceed these levels, obesity becomes more prominent. Agras goes on to caution practitioners to employ the lower end of the range for taller clients and the higher end for shorter ones. Unfortunately, for individuals needing to reduce, putting goals in BMI terms is arcane (NIH, 1985). Consequently, in our treatment plans clients are told about their BMIs but track progress in pounds or kilograms.

JUSTIFICATION FOR TREATMENT

Excess weight has been correlated with a panoply of physical ills including arteriosclerosis, hernia, hypertension, maturity-onset diabetes, toxemias of pregnancy, gallbladder disease, low back pain, osteoarthritis of the hips and knees, dermatological problems, surgical problems, and more. And gaining has been said to be more dangerous than remaining overweight. Medical reasons proposed for treating the obese are not only that doing so may reverse the course of some of these difficulties but also that obesity itself lowers life expectancy, is an independent risk factor of several diseases, exacerbates some already present health problems, and if alleviated may change risk factor profiles.

Measuring obesity in terms of relative weight, life insurance studies indicate that as overweight increases so does the mortality ratio. And when obesity is severe, longevity is markedly affected (NIH, 1985)— disproportionately so compared with lower levels of excess. Losing weight can perhaps improve one's chances of survival (NIH, 1985). If unrelated to any current or past illness, having a weight below the mean—at least 10% below the U.S. average (Manson, Stampfer, Henne-kens, & Willett, 1987)—may be best (lowest mortality), but very low (25% or more below average) apparently causes the mortality ratio to increase again (NIH, 1985).

Of Physical Well-being

Equally meaningful to health professionals, perhaps ultimately more basic and informative than determining survival ratios, is disclosing the relationship of overweight to disease—manifesting disease risks or actu-ally contracting illness. Reporting on the association of overweight and hypertension—blood pressure of at least 160 systolic and/or 95 diasto-lic—Van Itallie (1985) states:

> The relative risk of hypertension for overweight American adults aged 20 to 75 years is threefold that for the non-overweight. (p. 985)

The connection is especially strong for younger subjects, those under age 45; for them, prevalence is over five times higher for the overweight compared with the non-overweight (NIH, 1985). And weight loss ap-pears to possess an anti-hypertensive effect, lessening what Messerli (1984) calls the double burden of obesity and high blood pressure on the heart.

Paralleling findings on excess weight and hypertension, though less dramatic, are those of excess weight and hypercholesterolemia—serum cholesterol greater than 250 mg/dl. Again, the overweight young (20 to 44 years) appear to be worse off (Van Itallie, 1985). For the 45 years and over group, being overweight does not alter the chance of having high cholesterol.

When the lipoprotein carriers of serum cholesterol are studied (e.g., Garrison, Wilson, Castelli, Fenleib, Kannel, & McNamara, 1980), high levels of low density lipoprotein (LDL) cholesterol seem to be correlated with coronary heart disease. But high levels of high density lipoprotein cholesterol (HDL) appear to lessen the danger (see Rhoads, Gulbrand-sen, & Kagan, 1976).

Weight reduction may impact propitiously on these lipoprotein levels (Follick, Abrams, Smith, Henderson, & Herbert, 1984). Follick and col-leagues, to exemplify, investigated the impact of losing weight on the plasma lipid profiles of 42 overweight women. Significantly, these au-thors looked at both immediate post-treatment and long-term effects. Recommending a 1200 calorie diet, they gave the women a ten-session behavioral package, followed by a four-session program of maintenance teachings. In addition, they scrutinized their patients' low density and high density lipoprotein cholesterol levels before and after treatment and then again six months later.

Losing weight had its greatest impact on lipoprotein levels at the final checkup. LDL levels decreased from what they had been initially. The HDL/LDL ratio, while not changing positively right after behavioral treatment, did so at six months. At this time, HDL cholesterol was higher than it had been pre-treatment. These findings, from long-term checks, are more positive than are those of Brownell and Stunkard (1981b), and Thompson, Jeffery, Wing, and Wood (1979), who reported that HDL cholesterol initially decreased in women at the end of behavioral treatment. Positive changes in the lipid profiles of men seem to occur earlier than those in women (e.g., Brownell & Stunkard, 1981b).

Considering diabetes, Van Itallie (1985) warns that the risk for overweight adults is greater than it is for non-overweight ones. Prevalence of diabetes—losing weight reverses deleterious biochemical effects of non-insulin dependent diabetes mellitus (NIH, 1985)—is nearly three times more. Likewise, according to Framingham study data, the overweight, more so than the non-overweight, chance having coronary artery heart disease.

Data from the American Cancer Society study on hundreds of thousands of men and women (Simopoulos, 1986) shows males more likely to perish from cancer of the prostate, colon, and rectum if they are obese than if they are not. Similarly, obese females chance dying from cancer of the breast, gallbladder, uterus, biliary passages, and ovaries. What's more, the severely obese woman runs a very high risk of endometrial cancer (NIH, 1985).

These and other data are compelling. They led the panel of the NIH consensus development conference (NIH, 1985) to advise that losing weight be part of the treatment plans for various medical conditions, including adult-onset diabetes, hypertriglyceridemia or hypercholesterolemia, hypertension, gout, coronary heart disease, and chronic obstructive pulmonary disease. The panel warns those 20% or more over the desirable weight norms (according to Metropolitan tables) to reduce. Such caution is even stronger for the extremely overweight because, as the panel says, losing weight for them may be "lifesaving."

Sites of Fatness

Not only may degree of overweight (expressed in relative weight or BMI values) have health implications; so also may body fat distribution—how fatness is apportioned. Site of fat deposition, in other words, may be a risk factor in foretelling disease. Of particular importance is abdominal obesity or central fat distribution (see Donahue, Abbott, Bloom, Reed, & Yano, 1987; Garn, Sullivan, & Hawthorne, 1987).

The condition is diagnosed by measuring the ratio of waist to hip circumferences (WHC), where the waist dimension exceeds that of the hip. This "apple shape" male pattern is contrasted with the seemingly less hazardous female pattern of fat distribution, "the pear shape," of femoral and gluteal fatness (Jones, Hunt, Brown, & Norgan 1986). Abdominal fatness may be dangerous not only for men but also, when the WHC ratio is equal to or greater than approximately .8, for women, too (Bjorntorp, 1985).

Certainly not every overweight individual is on a collision course with illness or premature death (see Wooley & Wooley, 1984). The above discussion on medical risk deals with probabilities based on groups. Also, the presence of medical risk is not the only justification for offering treatment (Brownell & Foreyt, 1985).

Of Psychological Well-being

Indeed, as Brownell and Foreyt point out, psychological reasons for reducing are legitimate, too. They usually involve, at the outset, individuals' feeling badly about their obese bodies and chances in social situations. For many, rational programs for losing weight are therapeutic experiences.

Clearly, though, there are those seeking weight-loss treatment ostensibly for cosmetic reasons who should be counseled against doing so (see Polivy & Herman, 1985; Wooley & Wooley, 1984). For instance, a 19-year-old woman studying to be a ballerina sought my assistance in reducing—she wanted to lose ten pounds. In her words:

> I feel fat. My breasts are too large. I've even thought about a mastectomy, but I guess no one would give it to me. Right? (I nodded.) My teachers at the school (dance school) think I'm too fat, too. I need to lose, so that my dance gets better. I know I lost the part I wanted. It went to (name) who is thin. I guess I love to eat.
>
> A few times a week I buy a whole bunch of food like candy, chips, and smoked meat and eat until I feel like I'm going to pop. Then I make myself lose it—you know bring it up, but I guess I'm too late 'cause some of the calories stick.

In addition to bingeing and purging, this young women had had bouts of anorexia, where her weight had dropped alarmingly. Significantly, her network of friends and teachers validated her self-perceptions of being too fat. I encouraged her to see me for her eating and other difficulties, but she rejected the offer. I then told her I'd list names of other therapists nearby who could and would address these issues; she rejected that offer, too.

WHAT BEFALLS PROSPECTIVE
WEIGHT LOSERS

They do not have to look beyond the local supermarket to find popular magazines and tabloids that contain promises of no strain, quick-fix, permanent solutions for obesity. Television advertises weight-loss miracle devices as well. And in all parts of the land there are "diet gurus" claiming their programs are *the answers*. Indeed, weight-control hucksterism is rampant, for today reducing gimmicks and stratagems are everywhere. The weight-loss industry in the United States alone gets billions of the public's dollars annually.

There are nutritionally depleted food regimens, some frankly dangerous (e.g., Macrobiotic diet); extremely low calorie formulas; over-the-counter drugs containing the possibly harmful ingredient phenylpropanolamine (Fitzgerald, 1985); injections of human chorionic gonadotropin hormone (obtained from the urine of pregnant women); sweat-generating devices for the stomach; sauna suits; body wrapping to "'compact the fatty cells and free them of toxic fluid'" (Fitzgerald, 1985, p. 236); and more. Nonsense reigns supreme. The foolishness is there tantalizing the desperate—the vulnerable. Surely many of today's readily available weight-loss preparations and plans are silly and deceitful: if they do work it's not for the reasons the packagers cite—the special pills or foods one is asked to buy. Some are harmful; if they do work, it's not good that they have done so, for one is worse off for having tried them. Often the proposed solution lists a disclaimer, in small print, such as to be used with a 1200-calorie diet; or, as Fitzgerald (1985) notes about two exercise programs, a diet is unnecessary if the consumption of calories doesn't contribute to current weight.

As a result, Blackburn and Pavlou (1984) caution would-be weight controllers to be wary: be suspicious, they warn, of weight-loss promises (diets) pledging quick and simple answers and avowing single-food solutions. And be watchful of those plans that try to entice with assurances of secret formulas to bring on magical losses of fat—"No need to exert, no need to restrict."

Wanting a more sensible approach, the prospective weight loser may seek the services of a commercial reducing program, private or worksite self-help group, or weight-control specialist. As for the specialist, he or she will think of the individuals wishing treatment as potential candidates if possessing one or more of the following characteristics:

- 20% or more overweight
- overweight and demonstrating one or more risk factors of incipient illness

- overweight and already enduring some physical disease that is known to respond favorably to weight loss
- overweight and suffering from a weight-related burden to mobility
- overweight and despairing about looks and social handicaps

The therapy will probably involve food intake restriction (perhaps along with a pharmacologic intervention), exercise, and some form of behavior change teaching. It is the behavioral component—a well documented technology—with which this book aligns most closely.

BEHAVIOR THERAPY

Instances of some form of this technology for the overweight have been applied for over 20 years. But behavior therapy in obesity control certainly has had and continues to have its problems (Brownell & Foreyt, 1985; LeBow, 1984). I'll mention four I find particularly vexing.

Meaningful Losses

Too rarely are the weight losses presumed to result from therapy clinically significant. This is especially so for the individual having much weight to shed. Brief treatment, in which weight-loss goals are often under two pounds a week, is one reason for this deficiency.

Tracing the findings of behavioral treatment from its inception to the time of this writing, Brownell and Jeffery (1987), however, report that outcomes have improved. In earlier reports, end-of-treatment losses averaged about 11 pounds (Jeffery, Wing, & Stunkard, 1978). Now, some studies show drops in the 20 to 30 pound range. Perhaps, as these writers speculate, interventions are both better and longer.

Variable Losses

Results of behavioral treatment are highly variable. Some clients do very well. Some do not. And some even gain. Why there is so much variability and lack of predictability remains a mystery. An understanding of the patient by treatment interaction, which this variability undoubtedly reflects, is absent. Better procedures for matching client to treatment are needed.

Enduring Losses

Too rarely do therapists do more than just train and hope. This means that efforts to bring about abiding changes are needed. Training and hoping (Stokes & Baer, 1977) is failing to plan for durability. Behavioral researchers and therapists seem to act as if teaching overweight clients during the formal intervention phase of the therapy is sufficient.

Indeed, few workers in this area ever attempt to program continuing or lasting alterations by modifying what seem to be the critical actions leading to desired body changes. Rarely are follow-through strategies seen.

Despite this deficiency, reported follow-up lengths have increased over the years (Brownell & Jeffery, 1987). Yet documentation beyond two years is still very much the exception. Practitioners therefore do not have a sufficiently large literature from which to find clues to engineer long-range outcomes.

For behavior therapy's future to be characterized by enduring change, Brownell and Jeffery (1987) recommend developing better screening procedures for giving clients what is best—fitting clients to the best interventions, developing ways to improve the losses at post-treatment, and developing ways to improve the strategies of maintenance. Encouraging vigilance at self-monitoring weight, as will be noted later, does perhaps meaningfully approach the maintenance problem, as do relapse-coping practices and keeping up therapeutic contact.

Knowing Why Losses Occur

Too rarely do therapists know if clients comply. Staying in treatment—that is, showing up for therapy sessions—does not ensure compliance with treatment directives. Better strategies for monitoring compliance are required.

In addition, too rarely do therapists understand the relationship between the behavior and energy modifications they encourage and the body differences that result. Better assessment of behavior, energy, and body changes (e.g., in weight, in fat, in insulin sensitivity, in blood pressure, in blood lipids) will facilitate tests of this relationship (see above; Stalonas & Kirschenbaum, 1980).

Finally, too rarely do therapists make the fine-grain analyses required to describe what happens to clients who work through the treatment plan. Both successes and failures have to be examined (Barlow, Hayes, & Nelson, 1984).

IMPROVING OPTIONS

Taking the position that therapy for the overweight is, except for those who are dangerously heavy, of questionable merit, Wooley and Wooley (1984) argue more for treating obsessions concerning weight than for attempting to bring about weight loss itself. They view society as loudly anti-fat, and they feel that treating obesity expresses this antipathy more than it successfully eradicates a malignant condition. For the Wooleys, the targets of therapy should be self-recrimination and self-abusive patterns of eating induced by dieting (e.g., bingeing and purging) traceable to a thin-crazed culture. In their words:

> Weight change may, in some cases, be a worthwhile and attainable goal, but it cannot be the major goal of treatment and its appropriateness and feasibility can only become apparent as other problems are corrected. (p. 191)

They go on to suggest that once these perhaps more basic difficulties are solved, the person's desire to reduce may well lessen.

Such arguments are persuasive. Certainly there are many overweight who should be treated for their body-image disparagement and nonassertiveness. And there are overweight individuals whose repeated failures to reduce make further attempts unwise. Counseling them to accept their circumstances is well advised (Brownell & Foreyt, 1985). Finding out who they are, however, may take several interviews and treatment trials.

Stunkard (1984) attempts to improve the overweight individual's options not by questioning whether or not to treat but by proposing a classification scheme that aims to fit the client with the right therapy. His system, albeit preliminary, could perhaps help diminish the population of treatment failures. Surely it's one step in the service of providing sensible aid for the many who seek body-shape change for medical, social, and psychological reasons.

Using data obtained from the National Center for Health Statistics, Stunkard (1984) reports on the numbers of adult overweight females in the United States (see Vital and Health Statistics, 1983). He then formulates a tripartite classification system that categorizes women (data for men unavailable) by amount overweight. It also identifies percentages within groups, and recommends what are felt to be the best treatments currently available.

For instance, mild obesity, as Stunkard calls it, is the most numerous category—90.5% of the obese sample. Women in this grouping are 20% to 40% overweight and often evidence fat cell hypertrophy; fat cell hyperplasia is rarer. Treatments of choice are dieting and behavior modification. Brownell and Foreyt (1985), modifying Stunkard's classification system, name the mildly obese as being those under 30% to 40% overweight and see them as "ideal for a program of behavior modification."

Fewer of the obese fall within the next of Stunkard's categories: moderate obesity. The 9% herein range from 41% to 100% overweight. Frequently they are just hypertrophically obese, unless near the upper end of the category, in which case they are likely to be hyperplastically obese as well. For Stunkard, the best approach to treating the moderately obese is diet and behavior modification under medical surveillance. He sees moderate obesity as especially problematic for therapists. Brownell and Foreyt (1985) recommend that patients in this category receive behavior modification combined with a very low calorie diet (see chapter 2).

Lastly, the third and least numerous grouping is severe obesity. Here are .5% of the candidates. They are both hypertrophically and hyperplastically obese and more than 100% overweight (Brownell & Foreyt, 1985). For them, surgical treatment is thought to be proper. Gastric bypass surgery is recommended if other, more benign therapies, have been tried to no avail (Brownell & Foreyt, 1985).

THE DESPAIR OF BEING FAT

Numbers of the overweight, but certainly not all, undergo the rigors of disease, demonstrate defined risks (e.g., high blood pressure) of acquiring disease, or experience the bodily discomforts of excessive weight. Likewise, numbers of the overweight, but not all, suffer the despair accompanying the circumstance of being obese in our North American culture. Our society condemns fatness.

This condemnation is usually taken personally by those experiencing it. The derision engenders a desperation to be thin that makes the overweight vulnerable to the many readily available unscientific nostrums (see above) that trade on their desires for thinness. Because of pervasive and prolonged antipathy in which society stigmatizes the obese child, adolescent, and adult as characterologically weak, irritating, and ugly (DeJong, 1980; Edelman, 1982; Lerner & Korn, 1972; Louderback, 1970; Richardson, Goodman, Hastorf, & Dornbusch, 1961; Staffieri, 1967), many of the obese feel loathsome. What's more, often they themselves disparage the obese they see (LeBow, 1986) and feel responsible for being overfat (see Allon, 1980; Cahnman, 1968).

I'll try to illustrate how being on the receiving end of prolonged anti-obesity sentiment feels by offering a retrospection from one of my clients, a 30-year-old woman who currently is undergoing treatment. Note the multiple problems she experiences that require attention—a common occurrence. Note also how she weaves her obesity into the fabric of her life—it is, for her, an aspect that colors nearly everything. In her account, she expresses her emotions about her obesity and the life situations she traces to it:

> I have always been a very sensitive person, which does not help someone who is obese. As a child and teenager, obesity made me an introvert. I lived in fear of comments from the other kids and people in general. I would wear a girdle under my gym shorts when in exercise class and just about

died doing them (the exercises). I lived in horror when we would line up to be weighed. I would try to get out of it.

I used to get very upset when on my father's visits home (he worked in another locale) he would comment about my weight and scream at me, saying his sister thought I looked grotesque. Mom was supportive of me usually, but she too went through angry periods about my weight and would come home and chastise me for what I was eating. She always overfed us kids—treats were always in the food camp. I became a sneaky eater. I always wanted to eat by myself, so nobody would know. I have one sister and, even though she was and still is big, she always made fun of me. Now she'll say things like "that dress looks good on a person your size" and "your husband would like you better if you lost weight and were more attractive."

I spent two years in a brace to straighten my legs, so exercise was limited and I gained lots of weight before my gallbladder operation. As I mentioned, I detested going to the doctor, horrified he would weigh me. Twice so far I've lost weight in my life. It made me feel better about myself.

She goes on in her outpouring of sentiment to discuss her marriage and early adult years.

The first few years of my marriage involved abuse in the home. My husband hated me for being fat and was embarrassed to take me to (his occupation) functions. I couldn't attend dances, outings, or visit him at work. I really resented this. On the one hand I felt I deserved what he did, but on the other I was angry that someone was doing this to me. I felt I had no control over what happened.

Sex was horrible at that time because if it didn't go right, I'd get struck. For a long time I couldn't have sex because I was too frightened. I felt alone, trapped, depressed. I wanted to die—to me it was a way out.

When I didn't have periods the doctor told me I was too fat to have one! I was terrified of a gynecologist because I heard they weighed you in the office. So, I wouldn't go.

A few years after I got married I injured my knee. Things were still horrible with (husband). My knee sometimes would give out and I'd fall. Sometimes when this happened (husband) got mad at me because I couldn't get up—guess I disgusted him even more; once he kicked my bad leg. I went to several doctors about my knee—couldn't bend it. They told me it was because of my weight and if I didn't lose I'd be crippled in a wheelchair.

At the time all this was going on I was gaining a lot of weight and wrecking my knee further. Wound up in the hospital. The nurses made me feel like a blimp. Everything was an effort for them because of my size. Hospital gowns weren't big enough and all the so-called specialists said was that if I lost weight all my problems would stop.

It was during one of her hospitalizations for her knee that she entered therapy with a local psychologist and began to deal with her self-hatred and her husband's battering.

Finally I went to (name of hospital) and I met Dr._____. During my first session with him, I poured out my frustration at myself, the abuse, the way doctors and nurses made me feel, and my not being able to have a child. In therapy I realized I had to start drawing self-esteem and stop being dependent on others. I still had times I felt suicide was my only alternative, but in a while I learned better. I started learning about my feelings and ways of venting emotions. I blamed everything wrong in my life on my obesity and on others' reactions to it. But I stopped feeling so helpless and more in control. We all have responsibility in taking charge and making change for the better possible.

During this time, my father had a severe heart attack, but while he was getting better he began to really talk to me as an equal—finally he gave me some approval. But my mother and sister said I didn't handle his heart attack well.

I still have a lot of conflict, fears, and anger about my weight but after four years with Dr._____ I'm able to draw on the tools I was taught. My husband went through some of the therapy, too, and he reduced the abuse, though my weight still embarrasses him.

A while ago, Dr. (the therapist) moved to a new locale and referred this client to me.

Last Easter Sunday he (husband) abused me again and all the old fears have surfaced again. To leave this marriage, being the size that I am, would mean being alone. I don't delude myself that men would be breaking down doors to date me. I guess I'm losing confidence again. I have failed to get jobs because of my weight. So, I'm scared to stay married and scared to leave. Also, I love (husband). The one positive thing is I refuse to revert to old habits, like blowing my diet because I'm upset. One thing I'm learning with you is I can control, and controlling is something I think of as for me. At this point in time I'm tired of having to work on me for him (husband) and the relationship. My husband needs some further behavioral changes.

Major objectives in this client's therapy are helping her take steps to increase feelings of self-worth, extricating her from physical abuse, and losing weight. She vows that she will bring in the police if there are any further episodes of violence in the home. Her husband refuses offers of therapy. She now verbalizes clearly that she wants to reduce for herself.

The bulk of my narrative in ensuing chapters is about rational treatment. I'll talk of the condition of obesity but I do not wish to imply that obesity is by definition repugnant. I agree with such organizations as the National Association to Aid Fat Americans that support the idea that various body shapes should coexist in our culture. And I agree with writers who are outraged by society's maliciousness towards the fat. Also, as noted, I'm cognizant that sometimes one's desire to become thinner is so ill-conceived that therapy needs to target the specious reasoning. Surely, many of the overweight need help in setting more achievable goals for themselves.

Nonetheless, I find in my own clinical practice that I do sympathize with many who wish to remove the disadvantages of being fat that they see, hear, feel and endure. They have a right to ask for and receive help that is aimed at sensibly altering body shape. And after frankly discussing with them what obesity therapy is and is not—it's no guarantee of thinness—I'll make it available.

Two

Components and Strategies
of Therapy

This chapter names and discusses the building blocks of the interventions for the overweight. These components of treatment are packaged in various ways, depending on what clients require. A few of them, such as self-monitoring and stimulus control, do seem to be nearly always part of the overall treatment plan.

Practitioners err when they just presume that a client's failure to reduce after having tried one method or some package of them is the result of not adhering to the rules of application. Failure to lose or maintain the loss, as pointed out, could well be the result of a non-program physiological variable, such as metabolic rate adaptation or fat-cell hyperplasia. Obesity is a multifaceted condition affected by social, psychological, and physiological factors. One cannot realistically assume that it is entirely the outcome of learned behavior or the failure to learn certain behavior. Nonetheless, the procedures derived from operant and classical conditioning as well as cognitive behavior therapy—three of the areas from which most of the procedures named herein come—are applicable to treating it. They can become extremely valuable for the client.

For me, an overriding guideline in training professionals is my belief that therapists are best able to help the overweight when able to tailor care, and they are better able to tailor care when they understand and are flexible in using treatment's ingredients. I will be especially concerned with those practices useful in carrying out the program explained in the final five chapters.

The history of the behavioral control of obesity has been mainly the attempt to control eating by applying overt and covert conditioning tactics. A problem has been that many researchers and practitioners have conjectured, not proven, that the eating behavior of the overweight is distorted—that eating style is askew. The attitude has been, and for some still is, that if the overweight learn to eat like the non-overweight do they'll come to look more like the non-overweight (see Mahoney, 1975), a dubious assumption. Mahoney argues against it. He feels that the assumption gains status as truth, so long as we continue to attribute value to strategies for modifying eating without measuring their direct effects.

The classic account of the behavioral control of obesity, providing its logic, was Ferster, Nurnberger, and Levitt's (1962) exegesis. It gave rise to Stuart's more pragmatic and replicable reports (Stuart, 1967, 1971; Stuart & Davis, 1972), which in turn spurred an ensuing avalanche of interest. Stated and tabulated in most of these studies was weight loss, not eating behavior. In other words, these studies targeted body shape, not behavior. The supposition has been that weight reduction is the product of preceding actions. But as noted, early studies, as well as a number of later ones, say far too little about which behaviors cause which changes underlying weight loss. Be that as it may, the techniques in many of these reports are useful in tailoring comprehensive therapy for the overweight. A practical discussion of these methods follows.

PROVIDING CONSEQUENCES
FOR SPECIFIC ACTIONS

The building blocks of intervention under this rubric derive from the principles of operant conditioning. Each seeks to alter an event's future probability, most clearly expressed as change in frequency or rate.

Positive Reinforcement

First and foremost is positive reinforcement. As one of two methods for strengthening behavior, the other being negative reinforcement, positive reinforcement is following an event by a consequence that affects the event's future likelihood. For example, in one of the earliest attempts using learning principles to treat obesity, Moore and Crum (1969) targeted weight loss for strengthening. To accomplish their objective they applied praise, often an extremely powerful consequence. Even though weight loss per se is not a behavior, the authors were successful in their aim—through praising weight loss, they may have inadvertently strengthened actions culminating in it.

Their client, diagnosed chronic undifferentiated schizophrenic, was in her mid-twenties and resided in a mental hospital. She was believed to overeat—pre-treatment weight about 168 lbs. Past dieting attempts had been unsuccessful. After establishing praise's value to the client, the authors then simply approved daily of her weight losses and disapproved of her gains. They continued this simple manipulation for five months, and the woman lost 35 lbs. She had a minor relapse after the positive reinforcement procedure was temporarily discontinued but overcame it when the procedure was reapplied. Later, treatment was stopped again, but this time she held her ground. Perhaps, as Moore and Crum speculate, the reinforcement package helped her acquire self-control. Without information on the behavioral skills she mastered, one can't say for sure.

Bernard (1968) gives an even earlier illustration of positive reinforcement for the overweight. Here, as before, it was the main tactic. And here, as before, it was applied just to weight change. Bernard's client, like Moore and Crum's, was diagnosed schizophrenic and lived in a psychiatric hospital. She weighed 407 lbs.

Funds were made available to her for reducing. She could use them to buy such non-food items as dance tickets. Ten tokens were given for each pound shed, and weight checks were thrice weekly. She also was put on an 1800-calorie diet, which eventually was reduced to 1000 calories. In 20 weeks she took off 89 lbs.

As said, Bernard used tokens when aiding his client. Tokens are intermediaries to other, backup reinforcers (dance tickets). Earning them or points is an efficient way to allow clients to access a variety of enjoyable recreations (movies, music, reading). Other particularly useful potential positive reinforcers in weight control programs are money, jewelry, paintings, praise, approval, and other verbal feedback. Developing a list of personally valued outcomes is helpful. Cautela's (1977) reinforcement survey schedule and more open-ended interviewing are useful in finding clients' reinforcers.

Today, practitioners are less likely to put exclusive reliance on positive reinforcement as the only treatment. Its major use is adjunctive, sometimes as part of a contract (see below) that focuses on measurable changes in eating and activity. The likelihood that positive reinforcement will be efficiently used increases when the following rules of administration are held to.

Administer Contingently. The client should understand the explicit relationships between designated changes and consequent events. Each contingency is to be clearly stated as soon as it is put into effect. Accordingly, if a client, having difficulty planning a day's intake, is to plan just one of Tuesday's meals and one of Thursday's and then again one of Saturday's, the therapist must state precisely what daily compliance brings—perhaps points to spend toward an upcoming concert.

Administer Powerful Reinforcers. Even if powerful at treatment's start, by treatment's end consequences may weaken. Conceivably this could happen when it becomes harder to obtain the positive reinforcer. Losing weight, for instance, increases in difficulty as time passes, making the opportunity for reinforcement rarer. To offset this reinforcer-delivery problem, the payoffs for losing weight could be augmented over treatment. Thus, a dollar for reducing 1 lb at therapy's start could be doubled for taking off the same amount by the 30th week. Likewise, if a client tires of keeping food records, the payoffs for compliance could be enlarged.

Clients, as just said, are sometimes paid for progressing. How valuable these payments are to them at the outset is critical to the venture's success. Mann (1972) asked his clients to surrender cherished items (jewelry, medals), promising to return them contingent on weight loss. So did Jeffery, Thompson, and Wing (1978), who found powerful consequences to have dramatic results (see also Jeffery, Bjornson-Benson, Rosenthal, Lindquist, Kurth, & Johnson, 1984; Jeffery, Gerber, Rosenthal, & Lindquist, 1983; Wing, Epstein, Marcus, & Shapira, 1981).

In the Jeffery et al. (1984) study, 31 clients received ten weeks of weight-loss instruction. All quite overweight at the start, they were in one of four groups—three money-incentive conditions and a control. Reinforcement was earning back portions of a $200 deposit: $20 weekly for losing about 2 lbs (weight group), adhering to a stipulated calorie intake (calorie group), or attending sessions (attendance group).

The authors engineered good results by tying powerful reinforcers to either weight or calorie reduction. Their clients apparently did not take drastic steps to retrieve deposits. In contrast, some of Mann's (1972) clients did; they took diuretics and laxatives to promote reinforceable losses. Thus, in Mann's study, powerful reinforcers had an undesirable side effect.

Certainly, using powerful reinforcers is not bad practice. But when applying them, therapists should look at not only the magnitude of the body changes resulting but also how these changes are achieved. If large returns follow continuous weight losses and if continuing to reduce is hard to do (which often it is), positive reinforcement may ultimately be damaging.

Administer Sincerely. An originally powerful positive reinforcer may well lose its potency if given begrudgingly. Praise, especially, must be applied with sincerity. If given halfheartedly or overzealously, it's probably no longer praise to the client.

Administer Consistently. Consistent reinforcement, administering reinforcers for each occurrence of the event to be strengthened, is best overall. What's to be reinforced, the unit of behavior leading to reinforcement, should be sufficiently large to be practical but not so large as to be initially unachievable. Whatever the unit, avoid hit and miss reinforcement. Administer reinforcers consistently.

Positive Reinforcement to Initiate Behavior

The above principles can be used to not only strengthen events but also produce those that at therapy's start have a near-zero probability. Suppose, for instance, the would-be weight controller has never planned a day's intake or looked through and understood a calorie-counting book or, for more years than he or she can remember, exercised vigorously. These complex events would have to be built before completing them could be reinforced.

How difficult the building is depends on what's to be constructed and the client's initial skills. One tactic, modeling, has the therapist clearly demonstrating reinforceable, if imitated, behavior (e.g., completing a daily food record). Teaching steps are as follows:

1. State exactly what is wanted and the correct order of doing each part.
2. Demonstrate each part of the task separately.
3. Reinforce performance.
4. Progress only at the client's pace of mastery.

Another tactic, simpler albeit related, is instruction. As with modeling, it requires therapists to carefully and completely specify tasks and reinforce accomplishments. Praise combined with the client's own discernment of managing the self-help job are customary reinforcers.

Both modeling and instructing are often combined. For example, suppose the therapist and client agree on the importance of bringing exercise into the treatment plan. The client, a 36-year-old overweight man in good health—he's been examined by his physician—wants to rekindle his love of activity through brisk walking and light jogging. Let's say that since graduating college he's done little more than push pencils around a desk. As a recreation, walking combined with easy jogging appeals to him because it's simple to do. He realizes that his extensive travel schedule means keeping exercise equipment to a minimum—another reason to like the walking-jogging activity. The therapist tells him about and demonstrates appropriate warm-up and cool-down exercises and talks over the worth of the walk-jog-walk sequence (see Bowerman, Harris, & Shea, 1978). Walking is initially to account for most of the allotted fifteen-minute exercise period. Also demonstrated is using pulse rate as a guidepost of effort (e.g., Brownell, 1987). He is told, furthermore, not to overdo it, not to let exercise heart rate exceed 70% of maximum heart rate. Also, he is enjoined to consult a chart of optimal exercise heart rate values for his age (see Lindner, 1974). He's instructed to go easy but not so easy that he fails to move ahead. His goal is to increase exercise time to forty minutes daily, five times weekly. To pace advancement in the program, he could be helped to develop a self-rating form of perceived effort. Reinforcers for progressing could be therapist approval and client feedback from self-observed accomplishments.

Response Cost

Response cost is the flip side of positive reinforcement. Instead of attempting to strengthen an event, the attempt is to weaken an event. And instead of administering positive reinforcers contingently, the attempt is to withdraw them contingently.

For instance, failing to keep food records could cost a set amount daily or weekly; though there are exceptions, weight therapy transactions are often made weekly from a collection of daily records. Most likely, funds for the transaction are taken from pre-treatment deposits. Similarly, a client unable to leave refrigerated leftovers alone could be fined for sampling, for each "transgression." Of course, obtaining accurate reports of the event to be diminished might be difficult, especially if the fine is large. Clients in the natural environment have to want the help response cost is capable of providing, if it is ever to work.

Reinforcing Incompatible Behavior

Compared with the two procedures above, reinforcing incompatible behavior is probably less frequently employed. Still, it can be worthwhile in treatment. To apply it, a list of logical and desirable substitutes to behaviors interfering with progressing in the program is devised in collaboration with the client (see Brownell, 1987). When undesired actions are likely, the client practices an activity on the list; the activity supposedly produces its own positive reinforcement and thereby grows in strength.

Suppose, for example, a woman learning to plan, record, and analyze her failures at reducing is bothered, almost daily, by irrepressible urges to snack two or so hours before dinner. On her list of enjoyable substitutes is reading the newspaper or a science fiction novel. As a way to prevent or lessen snacking, she would be encouraged to try reading when snacking urges strike; the urge would be expected to dissipate soon. She would be told to save reading for these times.

The worth of positive reinforcement, response cost, and reinforcing incompatible behavior is, to repeat, adjunctive. In the therapist's arsenal of potentially effective intervention components, they can be arranged to fit the needs of the specific client. They are, however, best thought of as components of larger-scale interventions. As central treatments, they all are wanting.

CONTRACTING

A contract also is often adjunctive, but is itself a bigger part of intervention than the forenamed components. It's a way to supply clients with multiple aspects of therapy for handling either those problems apparent at the start of treatment or those arising later on. Notably, the contract, a signed document, is a clearly written agreement detailing an arrangement of consequences for doing and not doing stipulated actions. The consequences fuel the contract. They may be various items of value administered by the client or the therapist for observing the contract or withdrawn for not doing so. Typically, both of these practices, positive reinforcement and response cost, are included.

To illustrate contracting, I'll recount my experiences with a 32-year-old, 240-lb woman for whom it formed the basis of treatment. She underwent 47 weeks of therapy revolving around a system of renewable five-week agreements. Railing against long-term devices, she opted for consecutive short-term ones. They made goals seem reachable and success seem possible. Her first duty was surrendering $20 to me—she did this at each contract's start. These funds were returned for keeping food records, losing weight—two pounds a week—restricting calories to a set level, and exercising. They were kept for failing at these tasks and for not canceling sessions she couldn't attend. Forfeited money, with her approval, was sent to an organization she detested.

She signed seven of these agreements over the approximately year-long treatment, losing 53 lbs, which was 22% of her pre-treatment weight. Losses during the initial few contracts exceeded subsequent losses partly because of the later stress she experienced when suing her estranged husband for more child support payments. Even during this most upsetting time of her life, however, and to her credit, she only sustained a small relapse. In retrospect, I believe that I could have done more to help her directly manage stress (see Meichenbaum, 1985).

The contract attempted to reinforce not only weight loss but also such adaptive strategies as reducing daily calorie intake and increasing exercise, which culminate in loss. Had it only focused on lessening weight, there would have been a greater risk of her taking unwholesome measures to regain her $20—for her a lot of money.

With some clients, as implied, contracts that use powerful reinforcers for only taking off pounds may promote unhealthy stratagems. Recall Mann's (1972) study in which he had his clients surrender personal treasures to be earned back contingent on losing weight. Each of his eight clients signed contracts that specified the return of valuables for dropping in weight and forfeiture for not, or for gaining. Lengths of treatment varied and weekly reductions averaged between one and just over two pounds. As said, however, some of Mann's "successful" clients took laxatives and diuretics to reduce and thereby earn back their treasures.

Of course such methods, when routinely used, are unwholesome. In addition, when relied upon they preclude choosing and learning adaptive strategies. In brief, the wrong tactics are acquired. Why this happened to some of Mann's clients is difficult to say, but perhaps, as he discusses, his contracts "trapped" clients into either losing weight or losing out. After signing the devices, clients had to either comply with the weight loss imperative or lose their valuables. If the treasures were indeed treasurable, then the trap was indeed strong, increasing the chances some clients (especially those unable to reduce regularly) would attempt to wriggle free of it by behaving unhealthily.

Contracts vary in targets of change, reinforcers used, and frequency of transactions. Box 2.1 is a sample agreement. Note that with it, clients cannot earn back all deposited funds just for reducing or, for that matter, just changing one targeted action. A combination of events is needed.

Contracts also vary in running time. In the program of planning and recording to be discussed later, contracts are frequently brief therapy adjuncts for ameliorating newly found difficulties, for instance handling situations in which friends encourage eating. They are not time limited but event limited, lasting until the designated problems they are put in place for improve.

SELF-MONITORING

Self-monitoring—for instance self-observing actions or intentions—is a significant part of many treatment programs. For many of the overweight who learn to watch themselves, self-monitoring is illuminating, for it uncovers hidden connections between the environment and eating as well as the environment and activity. Indeed many clients are truly amazed by what they find from self-monitoring. The surprise signals a growing awareness about how their worlds impact on weight, and this awareness may in and of itself be therapeutic.

Through self-monitoring, clients may observe and record the types, quantities, preparations, and calories of foods. They may also learn to watch for urges preceding eating (Stuart, 1978a). What's more, they may

---

Box 2.1. Sample Contract

Name of client _____ Date of contract _____

Starting weight _____

Client Stipulates:

1. To finance the contract, which is to run for up to and no longer than 20 weeks, with the sum of $300.00 deposited with the therapist.

2. To lose at least one pound up to two pounds at each weekly weight check. Each week I fail to lose at least one pound from the previous week's weight, I will forfeit five dollars of this sum, and realize that I will be rewarded with five dollars for each pound up to two pounds from basal weight (see below) I do lose.

3. To control my daily calorie intake such that I do not exceed by 5%, or undercut by 5%, the daily allotment of _____ calories, agreed upon in session. For each period of seven consecutive days intervening between my scheduled visits that I do not exceed or undercut the recommended daily calorie allowance, I will receive $10.00. Each day I fail to live up to this calorie requirement, I will lose $1.00 and reduce my potential earnings by this amount from a total possible of $7.00. The extra $3.00 is a bonus for a perfect week. I recognize that daily calorie requirements may change over the time of the contract.

4. To follow the prescribed activity plan. For each period of seven consecutive days intervening between my scheduled visits that I meet the activity plan, I will receive $10.00. Each day I fail to live up to the activity requirement, I will lose $1.00 and reduce my potential earnings by this amount from the total possible of $10.00. I recognize that activity requirements may change over the time of the contract and that not always will there be seven days planned for. A week of activity, nonetheless, is defined as whatever my therapist and I agree to in session.

5. To be reimbursed for losing no more than 20 pounds from my starting weight during the run of this contract. Once this amount of weight is lost, this contract is void and a new contract may be negotiated. Also, once the entire deposit is earned back the contract ends, no matter if this circumstance occurs in less than 20 weeks.

6. To allow my basal weight to be set as the lowest amount of weight I have reduced to in any one session. My basal weight can never increase from my starting weight or any reduction that I achieve as measured during a therapy session.

7. To do my utmost to keep my weekly appointment. In the event that I am unable to arrive for my weekly visit, I will let my therapist know as soon as possible. If I fail to do this, I will forfeit $5.00. After two consecutive "no shows," therapy is automatically terminated and all monies deposited with the therapist are forfeited.

8. To allow my therapist to dispense any forfeited portion of the money I have deposited to the _____ provided I have not earned this back by the end of the contract period.

Patient's signature _____

Therapist Stipulates:

1. To pay the amounts designated for the weight losses and actions listed, up to but not exceeding the total amount of funds originally deposited.

2. To reimburse, when forenamed criteria are met, weekly.

3. To provide what is currently believed to be a rational and workable approach to overweight.

4. To dispense all forfeited monies within one week subsequent to the end of the contract.

Therapist's signature _____

track feelings, fatness, and pounds as well as daily activities, recreations, and the situational accompaniments of each repast.

To assess eating before therapy commences, clients observe immediately after having a meal. Forms for doing so abound (See Agras, 1987; Jeffrey & Katz, 1977; Jordan, Levitz, & Kimbrell, 1976). Box 2.2 portrays a simple one that functions as a preliminary record of eating, feelings before eating, and behavior surrounding the consumption act. Therapists look up calorie data after forms are returned.

To assess eating during therapy, clients could observe and record what they intend to consume a day or so before the meal or closer to it (see box 6.1) or what they have already in fact eaten (see box 6.2). Like ingestion, activity also may be planned, recorded after the fact, or both (see table 6.1). A client may monitor such activities as sleeping, taking the elevator, taking stairs, dressing, and watching television, as well as ones such as swimming, dancing, jogging, walking, or playing tennis. Time and effort would be estimated and translated into energy used. Thus, there is much the client may observe.

As implied, there are basically two reasons for self-monitoring: gathering assessment data for the practitioner to advise on treatment, and treating per se by producing data that cause the client to take steps to lose weight.

About the self-change possibility, a tentative explanation for it is that self-observation allows clients the opportunity to evaluate behaviors against self-imposed norms of appropriate action. Having knowledge of actual behavior and their own standards, they then decide whether to reward or punish themselves for what they've done, affecting by so doing their future pursuits (Kanfer, 1970, 1977; McFall, 1977).

For example, an overweight woman vacationing from work may observe and record taking 16 chocolates from a well-stocked living room candy dish and be appalled by what she has done. She sees her actions as markers of sheer gluttony and proof of her inability to lose weight. Because she thinks of her unplanned eating as discordant with her standard of behavior, she verbally castigates herself. In the future, she avoids going into the living room, or perhaps does read there but doesn't sample from the dish. Aware of shunning the candy, she possibly feels better about herself and lessens the probability of further unplanned eating.

The two reasons for self-monitoring, assessment and modification, sometimes conflict because of the technique's potential reactivity: monitoring can itself change what's monitored. Accurate assessment is less likely because of reactivity. Yet this behavior change effect of self-monitoring may rapidly dissipate, limiting its use as a sole treatment. Nonetheless, as part of a comprehensive therapy, self-monitoring is indispensable.

Box 2.2. Preliminary Food Chart
Fill Out Immediately After Eating

Name: _____

Date: _____

Unless instructed otherwise, do
not record calorie information.

Time	Feeling	Food	Qn.	Cals.	Activities Before	During	After

STIMULUS CONTROL

Stimulus control has been a mainstay of behaviorally based programs, but lackluster results suggest that it is nowhere near the therapist's supreme weapon—useful in therapy, no doubt, but it will not carry
the entire burden.

To explain the technology of stimulus control, let us consider the
environment and actions of an overweight male inveterate snacker. At
5:30 every weekday, he endures 30 miles of freeway traffic to travel home
from the bank where he's an officer. Soon after arriving at his residence,
while waiting for dinner, he'll eat chips, corn chips, pretzels, nuts—whatever he finds in the "snacks" cupboard, which he daily checks thoroughly.
Then he heads for the downstairs bar to enjoy light beer. Finishing, he
goes to the den, turns on the television and, while watching, snacks
more; this time he does so on hard candy that is prominently displayed
in a nearby dish. Later, within an hour and a half, he has a nutritious
dinner. Monday through Friday this sequence unfolds.

The problem with it is that this fellow is fatter than he wants to be.
The before-dinner sequence may be doing a lot to keep him that way.
Understanding stimulus control is, to a significant degree, understand-
ing the sequence.

Realize that this or a similar regularly occurring succession of eating
events is not something that confronts only the overweight. There are
many non-overweight snackers, too, but if one is fat chances are such
routines are hazardous. They exemplify how operant behavior can be
under antecedent control, stimulus control. Consequence control has
already been addressed in the context of using positive reinforcers, response cost, reinforcing incompatible behavior, and, to a great extent,
contracting. Antecedent control is in fact ultimately and largely dependent upon consequence control, but in the obesity treatment literature it
is often seen as separate.

Stimulus control of eating is as old as the first effort to modify obesity
by modifying behavior. To wit, Ferster and colleagues (1962) felt that the
overweight were victims of control by too few of the right kinds of antecedents and too many of the wrong kinds. These researchers would not
be surprised by the antics of our snacker. They might say, when attempting to explain them, that because time of day regularly precedes be-
tween-meal eating it comes to cue the act, as does the sight of snacks in
the cupboard, watching television, and the visible candy dish. Indeed,
many therapists would agree and also point out that this banker's knowledge of snacks being in the cupboard and cool drink being available
downstairs is probably critical, too.

Most of us are influenced in what we do by times, sights, places, situations, and thoughts. The therapist's concern is capitalizing upon this influence to optimize clients' chances of losing weight. Sometimes this is done by telling them to make a number of face valid changes in their food worlds—stimulus control of activity is rare. At other times, an attempt is made to have them first identify problems stimulus control technology might ameliorate.

There are various rules to suggest (see Agras, 1987; Brownell, 1987; Bellack, 1975; McReynolds, Lutz, Paulsen, & Kohrs, 1975; Stuart & Davis, 1972). Among those listed here are some to establish seemingly adaptive control and others to eliminate existing problematic control.

Directives Establishing Adaptive Connections

1. Break for exercise, make a telephone call, bathe, or whatever is desirable at the moment, so long as it is not eating, when the urge to eat between meals strikes.
2. Eat at specified times.
3. At home, eat at a specified place and do nothing else there.
4. Eat with specified eating utensils: placemat, dish, and cup.
5. Before going out to eat, consider what foods are available and desirable at the restaurant where an outing is planned.
6. Buy food at the market when wanting to eat is unlikely.
7. Put away leftovers in opaque containers and when possible store the containers in the refrigerator. When there is too little to store, throw out leftovers on the plate (plate-waste). Ask family members to help clear.
8. Make taking seconds harder to do (and possibly keep food from sight) by filling plates from the kitchen, not from the dining room.

Directives Breaking Undesired Connections

1. Remove food from all rooms but the kitchen.
2. Most foods on hand should require preparation before eating.
3. Do not eat when doing something else that's pleasurable, such as watching television or reading. Make the act of eating a singular event, and do not contaminate it with other activities.
4. Get rid of snack foods. They should not be easily obtained. If eliminating them entirely is impossible (the family objects), designate who is to get what. Have companions keep their snack foods in their own identified containers.
5. Ask waiters, when dining out, to avoid serving bread before salads and entrees.
6. To lessen sampling, try to begin the preparations for subsequent meals after finishing previous ones.

PACING EATING

Directives to slow down the rate of ingestion are to numbers of therapists just more stimulus control directives. Originally, attempts to have individuals reduce their speed with knife, fork, and spoon were born out of notions that slower eating was not only better for you nutritionally but also thinning.

Thus, to Horace Fletcher, an overweight millionaire, our endowment of 32 teeth meant that we should chew each bite of food 32 times. He issued this wisdom at the turn of the century, warning "nature will castigate those who don't masticate" (Carroll, Miller, & Nash, 1976, p. 375). Taking his own advice, he did lose weight, but there's no proof that his increased chewing had anything to do with it. Years later, the Ferster group (1962), using operant conditioning logic, portrayed eating as a chain of actions that, for the overweight, occurred too rapidly. For the late Charles Ferster, the chain needed to be slowed.

Today, it is unclear whether the obese really do eat faster than the non-obese do or whether slowing down is therapeutic. In light of these unknowns, it is reasonable to question the value of having obese eaters slow down. Potentially a desirable outcome of doing so is that they undergo the motivating and confidence-building experience of self-control (see Stuart, 1967). Also, possibly, slowing down might result in consuming less (cf. Booth, 1980).

At the outset of treatment, clients could be asked if they see themselves as being fast eaters. They can check this out by monitoring when for them the meal begins and ends and, importantly, how often they are first in the family to finish it. If after self-monitoring they do wish to slow down, tell them some of the commonly used pacing directives:

1. Chew food more.
2. Cut food to be put on the fork or spoon into smaller pieces.
3. Interrupt the meal perhaps by talking more.
4. Put down the eating utensils after taking a bite of food.
5. Swallow food in the mouth before taking a new bite.

SETTING OBJECTIVES

The number and explicitness of the goals clients are asked to assign themselves depend on the type of treatment plan they are to follow. As with many behaviorally based programs, the regimen discussed in this book has clients designate daily calorie intake levels, exercise goals, food-intake goals, and more. Having clients set objectives may be therapeutic, but why this may be so is unclear. Possibly it is feedback from attaining them that is influential—feedback possible only after setting them. If so, then therapists should help clients arrange objectives that maximize receiving positive feedback: small hurdles are better than large ones in this regard, because they are more manageable and allow for signs of progress sooner.

Smaller hurdles may also be less disruptive to the therapeutic process. Ferster and associates (1962) worried, for instance, that having clients try to meet relatively large weekly weight-loss goals would be like having them try to work under conditions of excessive food deprivation. The deprivation, it was thought, would be so severe that it would eventually undermine efforts to lose weight. The argument was that because food is an extremely powerful reinforcer, conditions of high deprivation have to be avoided. If such conditions continue, the client will stop complying with treatment—will take steps to alleviate discomfort. Though logical, their warning is at variance with literature on short-term fasting, which indicates how well in fact total deprivation is tolerated (Stunkard & Rush, 1974). Perhaps it's not actual deprivation that is the biggest problem but perceived deprivation. Clients should not see themselves as being too deprived. Also they should not see themselves as too far behind their goals.

Small hurdles may be the most realistic kind to have. Brownell (1987) views goal-setting in terms of attitudes. For him, having unrealistic objectives spells future trouble. So he cautions potential weight losers to evaluate carefully goals of weekly weight loss, projected time to no longer be overweight, anticipated ease of dieting, and expected future as a thinner person.

COGNITIVE RESTRUCTURING

Many of the overweight begin treatment desperate to solve what for them seems to be an unsolvable condition. Their pressure, their desperation to succeed at the weight-loss game is overwhelming. That feeling may be so intense as to lead them, as has been suggested, upon paths of excessive self-denial and overzealous exercise, both of which help bring on failure. Along these paths they find no shortage of occasions to condemn themselves for what they do. And by castigating themselves for disobeying what are really unreasonable plans, they despair and self-recriminate, causing further transgressions. Such clients too often confuse controlled eating with unremitting restriction and controlled exercise with herculean effort. Coupling the extremes of self-imposed denial and fanatical exercising with the urgency to lose weight quickly, they become treatment casualties. They, by their own thoughts and actions, then portray themselves as weak, piggish, and lazy.

Articulating the cognitive pattern generating this self-abuse, while assuming that thoughts are central to the control of external actions, Mahoney and Mahoney (1976) propose that clients have to change the nasty things they say to themselves. So does Brownell (1987), who identifies such counter-therapeutic self-dialogue as telling oneself that it's just the diet that causes weight loss—when on it things work, when off it things don't—rather than anything having to do with personal efforts to reduce; telling oneself that progress has to come about right away rather than having patience and fortitude; telling oneself that the new treatment plan is really old stuff rather than appreciating its differences. Similarly, Stunkard (1985) identifies negative self-talk about objectives, cravings, excuses, and losing weight.

Negative self-talk is changeable by rehearsing positive self-talk. Mahoney and Mahoney (1976) recommend a three-part procedure of having the client record both positive and negative monologues, evaluating the appropriateness of the latter type to the situations wherein they occur, and praising efforts and progress in treatment.

Clients' negative self-monologues are frequently the byproduct of perfectionistic standards and all-or-none, dichotomous thinking (e.g., Brownell, 1987). For instance, going about dieting feeling that no deviation is tolerable sets the dieter up for despair. Transgressions will happen, and the client has to be able to recoup from them. Client standards need moderating. Maintaining excellence is rarely possible throughout the prolonged time it takes to reduce significantly.

As Marlatt and Gordon (1980) elucidate in their analysis of relapses, the way clients interpret slips from perfection may well determine whether catastrophes, such as prematurely quitting, occur. Clients, it is thought, can reduce the chances of becoming the victims of slips. They can reduce the likelihood of causing further harm to themselves after lapsing by learning to keep violations from becoming so personally devastating. Some weight controllers are helped by learning to anticipate high-risk situations, acquiring ways to deal with them, and practicing how to cope with actually risky circumstances as well as with the guilt "slipping" brings (see Perri, Shapiro, Ludwig, Twentyman, & McAdoo, 1984).

ASSERTIVE RESPONDING

The great value for the client of mastering assertiveness is learning to handle others who disrupt the weight control enterprise. Disruptors may be friends who insist the client join them in consuming some unexpected rich treat. Or they may be hosts and spouses who don't take no for an answer when proffering second and third helpings. Or they may be coworkers who insist on offering rides. There are numbers of potential person-obstacles to losing weight. Clients are taught to be assertive to better deal with them.

Assertiveness Techniques

Assertiveness is standing up for one's rights (Alberti & Emmons, 1970). Teaching clients to do so means teaching them to overcome inhibitions interfering with expressing these rights. Techniques involve the following:

Identifying and Articulating the Difficulty. For instance, a female client's exercise program may be thwarted by unexpected visits of well-meaning friends who take up the allotted exercise time. Learning to be assertive requires that the client analyze the disruption (e.g., when it occurs, friend[s] involved, feelings toward friend[s], reasons for visits) and discuss it with the therapist. Role-playing would ensue, with the therapist playing the disrupter's part and the client playing herself. Feedback follows. The goal is clarifying the difficulty; using a video or audio of the interchange is helpful.

Developing Alternatives. The client and the therapist work together to design effective alternative monologues. The client has to discriminate non-assertive communication from aggressive communication and both of these from assertive statements. For the woman in our illustration, the non-assertive is what she says (or fails to say) when the friend drops by and stays too long. Equally damaging, the aggressive would be hurtful and could result in losing friends. The assertive, on the other hand, would likely have the desirable outcome of permitting exercise and keeping friends. The assertive statement might be: "Hi! You caught me at a bad time. I was exercising. I've got to finish before Sally comes home. I'd love to talk to you after. Do you want to stay while I finish?" If the friend says no, "Okay, let's talk later when there's more time. I'll call you, okay?"

Practicing Alternatives. As before, but now having an assertive message to give, the client would play herself while the therapist plays the friend. Feedback about the content and delivery of the message—speech, gestures—would follow. Then it is useful for client and therapist to switch parts. Running tapes of the practice sessions and having the client rehearse monologues imaginally are instructive.

Trying Out the Alternative. When the problem situation recurs, the client is to apply the assertive communication, feeding back to the therapist the positives and negatives of so doing. Adjustments are made and encouragement given. The client is to continue being assertive in the identified problem setting and in new ones that present themselves. Learning by doing occurs as clients try and succeed.

DIETING

For many of the overweight, diet is, as Garfield laments, "Die with a T" (Davis, 1980). In its modern usage, the word diet, originally Greek for course of life or mode of living, means the selection of foods we eat . . . most often a temporary selection of them.

What's a good diet? The final word on that question certainly has not been written, but it is instructive to read what the Committee on Dietary Allowances (1980) has to say about fat and carbohydrate. The guidelines they offer are appropriate for the obese, particularly those demonstrating various disease risk factors.

> Total fat intake, particularly in diets below 2000 kcal, should be reduced so fat is not more than 35 percent of dietary energy. Since fat has the highest caloric density of the primary nutrients, a decrease in fat consumption can produce the greatest change in dietary energy. There should be greater reduction in fats containing predominantly saturated fatty acids, such as those from animal sources, than in vegetable fats containing predominantly unsaturated fatty acids. These simultaneous changes in amount and type of dietary fat would increase the ratio of polyunsaturated to saturated fatty acids. The Committee on Dietary Allowances believes that in view of the possible hazards of high intakes of polyunsaturated oils (Food and Agriculture Organization, 1977), an upper limit of 10 percent of dietary energy as polyunsaturated fatty acids is advisable.
>
> Intake of refined sugar should be reduced and complex carbohydrates maintained or even increased. Refined sugar (sucrose) confers no nutritional value other than as a source of energy and under some conditions is a contributory factor in dental caries. Dietary sources of complex carbohydrate often provide necessary vitamins and minerals and in addition are considered desirable for proper intestinal function.
>
> For many individuals a reduction in alcohol consumption would also assist in achieving proper caloric balance. These recommendations for desirable types and amounts of dietary fat and carbohydrate do not entail radical changes in eating habits and could be accomplished with the United States food supply. (pp. 36–37)

Dieting is something more than diet. Blackburn and Pavlou (1983) capture this sentiment when they name as important not only a balanced bill of fare but also exercising and behavioral principles. Dieting signifies action, to the success of which the methods espoused in this chapter are supposed to contribute.

Teaching about calories and figuring the magnitude of calorie restriction to impose are just two of the therapist's tasks when trying to alter the client's food intake. Another is correcting misunderstandings about foods and nutrition. Misinformation abounds. For instance, Mahoney and Jeffrey (1974) list mistakes ranging from believing meal skipping is good, replacing food with vitamins, and thinking milk should be drunk in unlimited quantities to considering beer as very nutritious, protein as non-fattening, and toasting bread as a major calorie-saving practice. Discussing and tracking nutrition is necessary to uncover and correct such errors.

When choosing a diet, therapists will find an abundance of possibilities. That there is an abundance means no one diet has yet been devised that for the dieter is *the* answer. Many published selections, such as the Stuart and Davis exchange regimen wherein clients count calorie equivalent exchanges, are useful for instituting *moderate* calorie reductions of approximately 1200 calories per day.

Similarly modest restrictions are possible by having clients engineer their own diets. The advantage of self-construction is diminishing the temporariness built into most diets. That is, clients can replace published, preconceived diets with foods that they intend from the start of treatment to keep using. Departures from customary choices can and do work, but at some point what is usual and readily available is what will be consumed. Therefore, rather than risk returning to an environment where selecting food and regulating portions are problems, perhaps it's wisest to attempt to correct this environment from the outset.

Severe Restriction

One departure from the client's usual fare that also includes a return to it is the very low calorie diet (VLCD) plus behavior therapy (see Palgi et al., 1985). The goal of the combination is promoting large and enduring losses. Although controlled tests of the blend are new, reports about it are not.

Indeed well over a decade ago, Lindner and Blackburn (1976), treating 167 adults, gave impressive clinical data attesting to its potential. The three-phase therapy applied was intense and prolonged and was carried out for different participants in different obesity centers. During the first block of sessions, clients were medically evaluated and received exchange diets as well as some behavioral teaching. During the next phase, the VLCD was begun, accompanied by more behavioral training.

But it was during the third phase that the main portion of behavior therapy occurred, starting when the weight loss period ended. Termination of the VLCD was contingent upon losing well. Refeeding took place slowly while food management methods, such as stimulus control, were tried. As the authors stated, "substantial weight loss and maintenance of weight loss occurred" (p. 205). The best of the participants were lighter on average by almost 45 lbs at an 18-month to two-year follow-up (see also Bistrian & Sherman, 1978; Wadden, Stunkard, Brownell, & Day, 1985).

Sampling 59 men and women (mostly women), Wadden and Stunkard (1986) recently reported a controlled study of this diet–behavior therapy composite. All their participants were markedly overweight—women more than 90%, and men almost 70%. A comparison of the three groups (the VLCD alone, behavior therapy alone, and the two together) revealed large post-treatment weight losses for all conditions. The combined group, however, posted the best scores—over 42 lbs shed in six months.

The impact of behavior therapy was seen at the one-year follow-up. All groups regained, but far less was put back on for those undergoing the combined VLCD and behavior therapy regimen. Compared to the VLCD alone group, who at one year could boast only about a 10-lb drop, the combined group registered a significantly, 18 lbs more of a change.

Behavioral treatment in the study included many of the methods discussed in this chapter. The two-month-long VLCD of 400–500 calories a day was a high quality protein diet of lean meats supplemented by potassium, calcium, and sodium chloride. Note that this diet differs greatly from the poor quality protein liquid regimen of several years ago that was associated with a number of deaths. The present VLCD was begun after participants received a one-month balanced diet of 1000–2000 calories (an intake level for both behavioral conditions as well) and was followed by a refeeding period. Medical testing occurred every other week during the VLCD alone and combined conditions.

Commenting later on this study, Wadden (1987) remarks about what happened to the VLCD alone and behavior therapy alone subjects. Those in the condition of severe calorie restriction had only transitory success. Not so the behavior therapy subjects. They fared much better. Although both groups sustained equivalent losses by treatment's end, follow-up after one year revealed behavior therapy's superiority. Possibly, as Wadden implies, slow losses in contrast to rapid ones are better maintained.

He also extols the virtues of joining these rapid and slow loss treatments, heralding the union as "good news for the 8 million Americans who are markedly obese" (p. 50). Agras (1987) seems to share his enthusiasm, listing five indications for currently applying the combination: the client is over 50 lbs too heavy; the client might well, by undergoing the VLCD with behavior therapy, avoid surgery (e.g., gastroplasty); the client has had surgery for obesity and is relapsing; the client has failed to prosper from behavior therapy; the client's weight problem is, more than usual, risking unhealthiness. Agras also cautions therapists applying the approach to make certain there is medical, nutritional, and behavioral backup. Indeed, profound complications may arise when anyone is placed, even for such limited periods as 2–3 months, on the VLCD.

A FEW WORDS ABOUT
DRUG TREATMENT

Physicians, as indicated, sometimes prescribe anorectic agents, such as fenfluramine, for their overweight patients. They do so to help them better follow diets and reduce. Published research (e.g., Abramson, Garg, Cioffari, & Rotman, 1980; Bigelow, Griffiths, Liebson, & Kaliszak, 1980; Ost & Gotestam, 1976) on joining such drugs with behavior therapy has as one of its goals enhancing the clinical benefits of the therapy the client receives.

As with VLCD by itself, it seems that giving clients fenfluramine by itself, an apparently non-addictive compound with few side effects, is a poorer practice than giving them just behavior therapy. But compared with the VLCD studies, the weight losses from the drug–behavior therapy combination appear to be less well maintained; in one study, clients did not even do as well as with behavior therapy alone (Craighead, Stunkard, & O'Brien, 1981) and did no better than with behavior therapy alone in two others (Brownell & Stunkard, 1981; Craighead, 1984). Investigating timing of fenfluramine introduction, Craighead (1984) showed that giving the drug after half of the behavior therapy program was over produced better end-of-treatment losses than giving it from the start. The advantage, however, disappeared by the one-year follow-up. When discussing her findings, Craighead warns against indiscriminate use of this medication. She suggests that it is unnecessary for, and may compromise the maintenance outcomes of, clients who are able to prosper from behavior therapy by itself.

Yet, as Agras (1987) speculates, its administration may prove to be valuable for those who at behavior therapy's start seem to do poorly (Craighead, 1984). More study of this pharmacologic agent's adjunctive value and that of others (e.g., the antidepressant Doxepin as used by Nutzinger, Cayiroglu, Sachs, & Zapotoczky, 1985 and diethylpropion hydrochloride as used by Rodin, Elias, Silberstein, & Wagner, 1988) is required.

EXERCISE

Having clients increase daily routines and recreations is a recognized component of today's obesity treatments. Not only does exercise per se contribute to weight loss, it may well improve the client's adherence to other of the regimen's therapeutic parts (Stunkard, 1985). Moreover, regularly exercising may help overcome dietary-induced drops in metabolic rate. Discussion of the type and value of exercise, as well as illustrations of typical exercise dialogue, will appear later.

Three
Introducing Treatment

What qualities should therapists treating the overweight have? Research is conspicuously silent here (Brownell & Foreyt, 1985). Logic and experience say, however, that in weight control, as in other areas of caregiving, good therapists are able to nurture, magnify, and broaden small instances of progress. They are seen by their clients as genuine, warm, and tuned in. Moreover, they are trustworthy, empathic, and alert—alert to opportunities for praising and giving corrective feedback. I recall one such opportunity. Animated and feeling quite proud of herself, a client entered my office with this account:

> Bob is leaving Janet, and of course that's terrible news. I've told you how close Bob and I are (her brother) and how much I love him. Now he's messed things up again. What about the kids—Bobbie is four and Jody is two? But guess what? After hearing about all this from Janet and later from Bob I didn't eat. You know in the past I would have.

Much of the ensuing session was devoted to discussing her unhappy feelings and to her real triumph of not letting them set her back.

Therapists also put a premium on the quality of the therapeutic relationship for promoting change, and they attempt to inspire clients by instilling confidence. They bring to the treatment situation knowledge of weight control basics, including nutrition, physiology, and behavior, or else they demonstrate a willingness to acquire these basics.

In the pages that follow, I'll attempt to align what's said to the program described in the next several chapters and the protocol of appendix 2. I'll highlight therapist–client discussion topics and communicate aspects of giving care to the overweight. Many of the currently available obesity treatments would perhaps deal differently with the issues I'll address.

When introducing treatment, client commitments are sought and therapist commitments are given. First, however, it is necessary to judge if the client will benefit from weight loss treatment and, if not, what to counsel. Sometimes the decision is not to treat; as said in chapter 1, that choice may be easy to make. At other times deciding whether or not to give weight loss treatment is harder.

For one thing, there may be preeminent difficulties requiring immediate attention. Then again, some of these other problems do abate when the client begins to take charge of the weight problem. For example, I'm currently seeing a 35-year-old woman who has gone through many crises since starting weight therapy. Her losses have reflected her handling of them. Entering obesity therapy nearly two years ago—ostensibly for a 16-week trial—she weighed 240 lbs. As the quality of her marriage and self-esteem have fluctuated, she has lost, gained, and lost—now a total drop of 70 lb. Ending her treatment after four months would have been inappropriate. For numbers of overweight clients, helping them take steps to control weight improves moods, just as taking steps to improve moods influences weight. Therapy sessions may be divided between weight reduction and other collateral difficulties.

My position on offering treatment is that I will try to provide it for most adults 20% or more overweight who request it from me. Admittedly I have sometimes made it available to those slightly less overweight, too, in hopes of giving them as well a sensible, rational alternative to the stratagems they have undertaken or are likely to undertake. Also, I will see children (LeBow, 1984, 1986) and adolescents.

INITIAL DISCUSSION TOPICS

Once a client is accepted into treatment, significant parts of at least one or two early sessions are set aside for clearing up misunderstandings and dialoguing about expectations. At this time, some will decide against embarking on the struggle to lose weight or they will choose some other vehicle of change, often the passive approach of obtaining diet pills or being hypnotized. Possibly the therapist is informed of this at the end of the session or by phone just before the next scheduled meeting. Reasons for dropping out at this juncture almost invariably include aversion to the active role requested.

Purchases

Clients are asked to buy calorie counters, or the practitioner can make them available. Kraus' *Calories and Carbohydrates* (1979) is excellent. Clients are to buy the most recent edition. Practitioners should themselves have a comprehensive listing, such as Pennington and Nichols-Church's (1980) *Food Values of Portions Commonly Used* to answer the numerous questions they'll receive about calories. Clients are also asked to purchase a food weighing scale—found in most drug and department stores—and a notebook (diary) as well as a few sheets of graph paper. For the data-keeping chores, I often supply printed forms. One advantage of doing so is helping organize records for easy review.

Success, Failure, and Cure

Clients want to know how much they should take off to be successful. When I ask them for their opinion, I often hear about desired losses and anticipated rates of loss far greater than this program strives for—indeed some clients fully expect to reduce as much as five or more pounds a week. Although the attempt to set weekly, program, and overall goals is done later when the weight chart is explained (see box 4.1 & appendix 2), I would now try to disabuse them of extremist thinking. Pointing out first that researchers disagree about the exact amount anyone should weigh, I would say that our program tries to pick a comfortable, realistic, and personally acceptable weight. What's more, unless a special diet is called for under physician management, we aim for a slow weekly rate of loss, about one or two lbs.

Clients are also informed, however, that it is rare for anyone to lose this steadily, week after week. Usually the curve of weight change is jagged. It is anticipated that losses will alternate with gains. Yet it is hoped that losses will either outnumber the gains or be of a greater overall magnitude—both more numerous and larger. If they are not, clients are relieved to know, we'll do our best to learn why and what can be done to improve the picture.

Important as is finding out about how much to lose, probably even more pressing to clients is whether you have "the cure." You don't. What you do have at best is a rational approach to treating obesity that for many does provide measurable relief. Rarely, as indicated, do clients reduce all that they want—all that makes them overweight—although it does happen. My response at this stage is: be hopeful.

Yet I will go on to clarify that nothing automatically works for every-one, forever. Neither is there a magical solution nor an enduring quick cure. Conveying my promise to collaborate with them to search for workable, efficient, and healthful solutions, I also communicate my con-viction that what is to be offered is a sensible alternative to being on the roller coaster of weight loss and to punishing themselves with hot dog diets, all-fruit diets, guilt diets, or worse. I inform them that numbers of individuals have been helped by this alternative—most have lost some-thing, a few everything they had hoped to lose. Some, on the other hand, have lost nothing at all or have lost and then regained everything. Failures, I point out, are most likely during the attempt to continue or maintain progress. I want to be clear about all this, so that clients can decide if they wish to undergo the program.

In return, I might hear that failure at any point in treatment or afterwards just confirms their suspicions . . . they're hopeless. A client might say:

> I've tried everything I've heard or read about. My friend Susan went on a diet herself and did it without a hitch. She's stronger I guess than me. I'm still a member of (local self-help group) and I go sometimes. Nothing works. Dr. (local physician) said he would call you about me. He said you're a behavior therapist and that behavior therapy is the kind of tough stuff I need. He also said you're a psychologist. Maybe it's my head that needs fixing. One thing's for sure: I'm weak—no willpower. Honestly, if you can't help me, I'm done. There's nothing else.

My response to such a message would have several objectives: to affirm that failure is neither *the* sign of a psychological problem nor the proof that there is not and never will be a safe, efficient treatment for obesity; to communicate that there are various physiological reasons for failure and more unknowns in explaining and treating obesity than knowns; to indicate that just because two individuals are overweight does not mean that they have anything else in common; to maintain now and later that unless medical reasons underlie the attempt to reduce, losing weight is born out of the desperation society instills to be thin, a reason needing evaluation and continued reevaluation. As noted, when faced with clients desperate to be thin and devastated by their repeated inability to be so, it is wise to try and counsel them to stop trying to lose and instead to try to stop gaining. For some, maintenance, even if overweight, is acceptable. Acquiring control over eating behavior, to someone feeling that this significant part of life is out of control, can be a wonderful achievement . . . even if little or no weight is shed.

Locus of Change

Localization of positive and negative changes is another, albeit related, issue repeatedly arising in treatment. Blaming no progress on a weak will, as just exemplified, is a source of much self-recrimination and defeatist thinking. Many clients, already expert at doing this, will not be dissuaded from it entirely. The following script, however, does help them explore the problems with such an internal, self-castigating explanation.

Well-wishers and guilt-mongers will freely give you this advice, 'just stop eating so much!' The advice smacks of the philosophy of increase your willpower. But eating or not doing so isn't something you can always just make up your mind about, that is *will* to start or stop. Eating is greatly influenced by many circumstances different from your will—circumstances apart from you, external to you. Sometimes, for instance, you eat without even realizing you're doing so. Or some kind soul gives you a rich treat and you can't say no without feeling that you're hurting feelings.

Don't be misled into believing that all it takes is willpower to handle these and the other obstacles standing in the way of your losing weight. Sure, there are people who, it seems, simply quit smoking or who, it seems, simply lose weight, but appearances are deceptive. These people have done something more than just make up their minds to conquer their problems. They have done more than just exhibit willpower. Exactly what that something is may be as mysterious to them as it is to you, but something good has happened. . . . some thing or things have changed for the better.

What is being said is that you're involved in your own change. Indeed, you're central to it. And I firmly believe you can take steps to be the architect instead of the victim of it.

What is being said also is that you'll increase the chances of doing well when you take stock of such actions as getting rid of snack foods from the kitchen or storing leftovers instead of eating them, or planning menus and exercises well ahead. And you'll take a step toward doing well when you take stock of what you say to yourself about dieting, being overweight, and being thinner.

What I want is for you to stop the self-recrimination. Stop damning yourself with the idea that you lack willpower. Lambasting yourself with the willpower stick keeps you ignorant of issues, actions, and thoughts that need your attention.

In your mind, distinguish willpower from responsibility. Willpower—or, rather, trying to explain why you do what you do in willpower terms—is passive accounting. Usually, it's looking for explanations in terms of internal weaknesses. You tell yourself that you do what you do because your personality or character is weak. Responsibility, on the other hand, is active accounting. It's looking for things to change, either such things as what you buy at the supermarket and the schedule you keep at work that keeps you inactive, or such things as the rigid diet standards you set up.

So, unlike the willpower search, the responsibility search is constructive. It looks for things to change, not for presumed and undocumentable character flaws. Explaining in willpower terms is fruitless, often demeaning, and detracting. It can blur the active, constructive search you need to make.

Triangulating the Problem

Clients are told to think of their obesity as multifaceted and to realize that obesity itself is not automatically equalizing: two people are not necessarily alike just because they both are equally fat (e.g., Kiesler, 1966). Relatedly, they are to think of treatment as multifaceted and best personalized. What's more, it is useful, they are told, to think about treatment in terms of a triangle. Each of the triangle's three points identifies a measurable part of the obesity puzzle. And each point influences changes in other points. Point A, the apex of the triangle, identifies body components, whereas points B and C are, in turn, for behaviors and calories—intake and outgo.

As for the top point of the triangle, clients hear, usually they've heard this before, that being overweight is different from being overfat. Yet often when one condition exists, so does the other. It is important for them not to lose sight of either body component. Greater information about discriminating weight from fat as well as about calories is presented later (see chapters 4 and 5). What is also mentioned briefly here, and again later, is the supposition that weight and fatness are the result of calorie balance changes brought about by behavior changes.

The therapist might say:

> There's a thin you and a fat you. You and I will have to keep track of both of you. That's part of the triangle describing you that is drawn on the blackboard. There's more to this point, point A, such as blood pressure and cholesterol, but for now let's just say that point A is for weight and fatness.
>
> Below that point is point C. That's for calories, calorie intake and calorie outgo. As a living person, you must take in calories and expend them daily. As you probably know already, if you take in more than you need for a time—and needs vary from person to person and from condition to condition in the same person—you'll get fatter.
>
> We feel that a great help in manipulating the amount of calories you take in and expend in order to lose weight and fat is altering conduct affecting calories. That means changing behavior, changing point B.

Numerous examples are given in conjunction with continued reference to the obesity triangle drawn on paper or blackboard.

Threats to Motivation

The next issue to identify, one related to much of the above and one that will very likely surface again and again, is client motivation to persevere and comply. As therapists and their clients are painfully aware, the eagerness of the first few days and weeks dissipates for clients, as required tasks seem to grow more burdensome and the rewards from doing them more trivial.

My objective is to introduce clients to three frequently occurring motivation-breakers. They may become the primary issues of later therapy sessions. Although losing motivation is by no means inevitable, I stress to clients that telling me about the decline when they feel it happening is vital. I want to focus on it in therapy. Fighting back against shrinking motivation is possible. Dialogue such as the following might occur at this time:

> *Therapist:* Right now you seem all set to go full steam ahead and try to lose. It's possible, however, judging from what I and many of my colleagues in this field see, that your motivation will decrease.
>
> *Client:* Don't worry, I'm not a quitter.
>
> *Therapist:* I don't mean to imply that you are. What I'm getting at is, things happen to people trying to reduce that make them want to stop trying. When these things happen—or, more logically, when you no longer feel that weight therapy is for you—let me know before you make up your mind to stop. I want what's best for you, and if ending weight therapy is best I'll support that decision. But early warning helps. It's possible that some loss of interest, if it occurs, is correctable, so we should try to make the corrections. Right?
>
> *Client:* Can you tell me about them? Maybe some of them happened to me the last time I tried losing and gave up disgusted.
>
> *Therapist:* Well, a big one that may arise soon after starting a diet is that rewards slow down and perhaps for a time stop completely, even though you do everything you're supposed to do. By rewards I mean regularly losing weight. What happens is that your body answers your behavior adaptively . . . adaptive, I should point out, if you lived where food supplies were low, but you don't.
>
> Let me explain. The rate you use up energy for living, that is for such basal metabolic processes as breathing, pumping blood throughout the body, and many more life supports changes because of dieting. In other terms, the old rate of using energy to run your body adapts to your dieting.
>
> That means it becomes tougher to get rid of excess calories in order to reduce. When there is a metabolic rate slow down energy is saved. This sort of saving no one wanting to lose weight is happy about. To picture its severity, realize that you spend more energy just staying alive than in any other way, including exercising. Not only are the basal processes the body's main draw upon its energy supplies, they're the first draw on them—life support comes first. To exist, men spend about a calorie of energy per hour for each kilogram they weigh and women about nine-tenths of a calorie. This figure varies depending on who is measured and depending, even in the same person, on physical shape, age, and other circumstances.
>
> As I've just said, one of the most critical of these other circumstances is dieting. After being on a diet for a while the amount of energy naturally used up each hour goes down, which means that continuing to lose weight gets harder and harder to do. It's as if your body answers you back when you diet by saying if you feed me less, I'll need less.
>
> *Client:* So it gets harder to use up energy?
>
> *Therapist:* Yes, I guess that's what I am saying. After starting to diet, for some people, it gets more and more difficult to burn up as much energy as they did before they started. But there may be something that can be done about this. There's evidence that exercising will help stop and

perhaps even reverse this drop in metabolic rate. One way to battle it may well be to exercise regularly. We'll talk about exercise in this program.

Client: Shouldn't I diet?

Therapist: I have to say that there are more than just one or two professionals advising against it. But I'm not among them when it comes to most of the overweight people I see. Certainly, though, I'm appalled by the diet-silliness that there is. No dieting is better than ridiculous dieting.

Client: I think you're trying to bring me down to earth with all this talk.

Therapist: It's not that so much as it's a desire to disclose fully. You're about to invest a lot of your time, effort, and concern in struggling to lose weight, and I want you to know what could be in store.

Another thing to be aware of because it can diminish your zest to continue trying is feeling abandoned while laboring to reduce. We'll talk about this at various times, but for now I'll just say that getting family and friends to help could be a morale booster. I say could be because a lot depends on your feelings about including others in this.

I also want you to be on the lookout for something else that may add to wanting to quit. Watch out for feeling that parts of the program seem wrong, feeling that for you the program misses the mark. Don't neglect telling me when you think this way. With your input, I can adjust procedures for a better fit or, if need be, remove them entirely.

KEEPING CLIENTS

Having already told clients this is an active program in which they, in collaboration with the therapist, will search for solutions, I'll seek a commitment to attend sessions. This step is to help reduce attrition. Dropping out is a serious problem; sometimes as many as 80% of clients starting treatment don't finish it (Brownell & Foreyt, 1985; Wilson & Brownell, 1980). Although behaviorally based programs do a comparatively good job of keeping clients (Brownell & Foreyt, 1985; Wilson & Brownell, 1980), attrition is still generally too high even here (cf. Eufemia & Wesoloski, 1985). Research about dropouts (see Bennett & Jones, 1986) is sparse.

Despite the deficiency, there are, born out of clinical experience, practical guidelines for keeping clients; some of these guides are related to what's just been discussed about motivation. The following are useful:

1. Solicit continued feedback about treatment so that those parts of it thought to be ineffective can be altered or perhaps purged. Clients believing that some requested changes are nonsensical may reject the entire package, even though a few of the components are deemed "worthy."

2. Help clients prevent treatment from causing family friction (see chapter 6).

3. Minimize mismatches if groups are to be run. If, for instance, a group of six overweight women commences with five being 22–33 lbs too heavy and the sixth being 80 lbs too heavy, the larger woman may quit, feeling separated from her colleagues in weight, attractiveness, and opportunities.
4. Follow through. When giving assignments, such as making food records, evaluate resulting data in the client's presence and praise efforts (Stuart, 1978b).
5. Exhort clients to come to sessions and from time to time restate the value of doing so.
6. Arrange deposit-contracts.

By taking several of these steps in his study of spouse-teaching, Pearce (1980) kept attrition to zero. He reinforced progress, made discussions lively, and fostered support. He also put a refundable deposit-contract in place.

The last guideline, arrange deposit-contracts, has been tested (Eufemia & Wesoloski, 1985; Hagen, Foreyt, & Durham, 1976; Sperduto & O'Brien, 1983). Hagen et al., in their classic account, evaluated the effects of monetary deposits on attrition. Before treatment, either some, all, or none of a previously requested $20 deposit was returned to the subjects. Two groups not having all monies returned were promised their funds for coming to 10 out of the 12 planned meetings, 80%. The three conditions differed in what they'd get for attending: $20, $5, or nothing.

Results were that much of the attrition was in the no deposit condition. The group standing to forfeit the most, the $20 group, lost only one participant. The pattern of mean weight loss, however, was the reverse. Those doing the best were in the group depositing nothing, those doing the worst were in the condition paying $20. Is it better to have higher weight losses and higher attrition or lower weight losses and lower attrition? As Hagen and colleagues point out, the two variables were negatively related. Attaching the monetary threat to quitting may have, it seems, constrained a few of the poorer weight losers in the $20 group to stay in treatment. Those in the no deposit group who happened to be poorer losers quit early. In brief, perhaps steps for lowering attrition kept unmotivated clients coming, and that's all it kept them doing.

Deposit-refund contracts could be arranged by the end of the first week such that funds from initial fees are set aside for being present for 80% of treatment and all follow-up meetings; only illness and catastrophic consequences would nullify either of these agreements. A $300 program, for instance, could earmark the potential return of $100—half for attending treatment and the remaining $50 for coming to follow up sessions. Even if program costs are negligible, the deposit-refund system is still viable. Clients could surrender valuables other than money. In our programs, wherein clients are primarily seen individually, we have effectively employed the deposit-refund system for encouraging attendance.

MEDICAL INPUT AND INTERVIEW

Years ago a psychiatrist and I offered a group of seven overweight men and women obesity therapy. After about six weeks we, and the group as well, began extolling the virtues of regular exercise. The real target of our pitch was a sedentary amateur chef who knew more about the calories in foods than anyone I have, to this date, met. Either because of agreeing with what we said or possibly wanting to shut us up, he took up the exercise gauntlet. Praise from all ensued. Then, one day, my colleague and I explored how this man felt about his new activity program. He informed us:

> I really think it's good. The only part I hate is going up the stairs fast. My chest hurts when I do it and afterwards. You know I had a coronary a few years ago.

We didn't know. We had him stop exercising immediately and sent him to his cardiologist. Clearly, we should have known about the heart condition before encouraging him to climb stairs. His response to our wonderment over his not telling us was, "you never asked." He trusted us to give him the right prescriptions. We trusted him to check our zeal. I still trust my clients to give me feedback about the consequences of what they do, and they, I believe, trust me to give correct, competent recommendations. But, especially at treatment's start, I no longer just simply wait for them to tell me about their physical shape. Early on, my coworkers and I ask each to have a physician complete the form in appendix 5 to alert us to dietary and exercise proscriptions as well as chronic ailments and other medical conditions. Also, during early sessions clients are asked questions about their health and current medications. The interview (see appendix 4) they receive is multi-sectioned and primarily open-ended. There are parts asking for demographic information, obesity history, eating and exercise practices, and problems perceived. Clients are usually asked to fill out at least half the interview themselves, but the obtained data are reviewed in their presence.

SOCIAL SUPPORT

It has long been recognized that the social milieu influences behavior, desirable and undesirable alike (Whittaker & Garbarino, 1983). Sometimes an effective informal support network involving relatives and friends, whose bond with the client is caring and continuous association, may already be in place.

Sometimes, however, instead of support there's sabotage. I recall a client whose husband, quite willing to pay for his wife's weight therapy, cajoled her into seeking such care. But he celebrated each of her triumphs by insisting they devour a gourmet meal—he willingly paid for that, too. He never listened to her protests and she never came near her goal weight. Over several months, she lost and regained the same few pounds. Despite my efforts and hers, he remained a saboteur.

Brownell and Foreyt (1985) offer plausible and interconnected reasons why spouses may do such things, among which are: fearing that the weight-loser will be sought after sexually; fearing that the weight-loser will precipitate lifestyle changes that alter the marriage or that suggest it needs improvement; feeling threatened by the weight loser's triumphs. Recognizing the difficulties, Brownell and Foreyt advocate including spouses in therapy (Brownell, Heckerman, Westlake, Hayes, & Monti, 1978; Pearce, LeBow, & Orchard, 1981).

Pearce et al. (1981) did test spouse-present vs. spouse-absent conditions in a diet plus exercise combined with behavior therapy package. He included also placebo and delayed treatment groups and articulated disengagement roles for non-cooperative spouses. Post-treatment differences did not significantly differentiate among the conditions. A year later, however, differences did emerge. The spouses-in-treatment group posted better scores than the client-alone one and also appeared to be continuing to progress, suggesting to Pearce that helpers impacted the most after treatment had ended.

The outcome hoped for when bringing significant others into the client's therapy is possible extension of its positive results. *Possible* is a key word, for to date the actual results of this practice have varied (Black & Lantz, 1984; Brownell et al., 1978; Brownell & Stunkard, 1981a; Dubbert & Wilson, 1984; Murphy, Williamson, Buxton, Moody, Absher, & Warner, 1982). Also varying is the choice of helpers—spouses, friends external to the family—and the helping roles assigned, such as reinforcing weight loss or monitoring record keeping.

Individuals whom clients would allow to act as helpers, individuals perceived as capable of rendering aid, are potentially valuable therapy resources. Locating them (the client may prefer to go it alone) is done through questioning. If clients do choose someone, I would invite the person to join us for preliminary discussion. The original offer to participate is usually made by the client. If the potential helper does agree to become an ally, I would ask for attendance at a pre-set number of treatment meetings, teach facets of the program, and with client input engineer rewards for efforts.

Four
Tailoring a Treatment and Involving the Client: Body Variables

The preceding two chapters addressed, in turn, frequently applied ingredients of therapy and introducing treatment. This chapter and the three following put together much of what's been said and, going a step further, lay out a tailored treatment, certainly not the only one possible. Clients most receptive to it are the mildly to moderately obese (chapter 1). Although the prognosis is less than sanguine for the severely obese, I and my coworkers have at times used it effectively for them as well. For instance, one of my supervisees treated a 26-year-old, 5 ft 10 in., 320-lb man who to no avail had tried reducing several times before. Faring better here, he lost, by the fourth month of therapy, 44 lbs. Approaching the second year afterwards, sessions becoming intermittent, he reduced to under 207 lbs—a loss of 113 lbs in 74 weeks.

He underwent a cover-best-bets regime that tailored prescriptions and proscriptions. It's distinguishable from the cover-all-bets approach, in which a large number of do's and don'ts are advised (LeBow, 1981). Our strategy is to search for the unique constellation of difficulties besetting each client and to tailor remedies (see also Mahoney & Mahoney, 1976). To uncover this constellation, clients plan to diet and become active, and then ascertain why they have difficulty doing so effectively.

The question is why can't the client sustain the weight loss regimen—sustain, for an amount of time varying with problem severity, a regimen of eating less and moving more? What are the roadblocks? Why is reduction so hard, which for us translates to the question of what contributes to violating straightforward plans to eat certain foods in certain amounts and to be active in designated ways. The process of answering is to have clients set goals and self-monitor the sources of every plan violation.

Violations comprise either rare or recurring behaviors with immediate

51

antecedents, sometimes identifiable consequences, and underlying sources (themes, obstacles). The client's role is planning food and activity schedules and searching for plan violations. The practitioner's role is collaborating with the client to encourage vigilance in making plans, and devising tactics to remedy bad planning as well as foster good planning. Much of this process is an assessment that spells out and polishes treatment.

In helping clients handle weight control difficulties, practitioners encourage a continuous refinement of the intervention which is closely tied to the specific reducing problems. Tailoring is a continuous, interactive process. To teach ways of dealing with weight control difficulties, the practitioner and client track weight and fat (size), energy, and behavior. Techniques for gathering data are taught at the outset and used regularly at first; then, as the client progresses, they are used intermittently.

As discussed, before beginning the program much of the process and several of the physiological and psychological pitfalls of obesity control are introduced. Client commitment is sought, and the realities of treatment stated. Clients are told that there are no guarantees of success, but what they are about to undergo, should they decide to, is a rational approach to living differently that for numbers of individuals has had desirable results.

A rationale of searching for and solving plan violations could be stated, such as the following:

> Remember our discussion of the triangle of obesity. I pointed out that to lose weight you have to shrink the balance of calories. But as you know that's not so easy. Why it's not so easy is not fully known yet. For one thing, there's the problem of basal metabolic rate adaptation and others that we discussed.
>
> Yet another problem, one I feel many people wanting to lose weight have and one this program focuses on, is living up to reducing plans. By that I mean plans to eat less and plans to exercise more—specific plans. My feeling is that you have to learn to plan effectively by finding out about the roadblocks preventing you from doing so. I'll have lots more to say about that in the coming weeks.

I would at this time illustrate what is meant by a roadblock. For example, letting someone interfere with the intention to eat less, and as a result taking in unplanned-for calories and feeling badly.

A 27-year-old, 249-lb client of mine, trying valiantly to follow his diet, exhibited this problem several weeks after beginning therapy. He writes:

> Went down the stairs (walked the five flights from LeBow's office) to Al's car. Nice he waited for me, but why did he have to go to (local fast-food restaurant) and buy so many french fries? He's even fatter than I am.

Waved the bag right under my nose and insisted I take one. 'One can't hurt,' he pressed. How could I say no? He's such a nice fellow.

I would let clients know that until we have the information about their own personal roadblocks, no methods other than the discovery method of self-monitoring will be applied.

TRACKING WEIGHT

In obesity triangle terms, we will now and for the remainder of this chapter consider point A (body) changes presumably induced by treatment. Appendix 2 puts the information in a stepwise format for operating convenience. Weight is foremost among the body variables clients love to track and practitioners find reliable and easy to track. The measurement is usually made weekly. More often is unnecessary and sometimes even undesirable, because when weight is assessed there may be no detectable loss. Weight change does not mirror right away the small alterations in living wrought from treatment. A lack of detectable difference after effort has been expended can negatively affect the client's mood, unfairly so when these absences belie propitious transformations in fatness (LeBow, 1977). Indeed, because of a temporary exaggeration in carbohydrate intake or because of times during the female client's menstrual cycle or because of fat loss itself momentarily masking weight loss (see Bray, 1976), clients may retain water and fail to register a weight loss when in fact fat has been shed. The weight check won't reflect this modification and therefore, under this circumstance, gives false information. Frequent checks increase the chances of clients receiving false information.

The best, most valid and more importantly most reliable, weight tracking devices are devoid of springs. Spring-type scales (the typical bathroom scale) display weights differently if clients move laterally when standing on them or if the scales are put in different areas of the same room. The mood generation problem of weighing frequently is compounded by an unreliable instrument, so advise clients against using bathroom scales too often. When they are employed they should be kept in the same place, with a mark where the toes are to go.

Expressing Weight Changes

To the client, the simplest and most meaningful gauge of weight change is pounds lost.

Pounds lost = time 1 weight minus time 2 weight

(time 1 is the initial assessment and time 2 later on, such as post-treatment.)

When used to compare heavy and light persons, this formula is biased against the light—the heavy do better—because those with more to lose have more available to lose (see Bellack & Rozensky, 1975). Practitioners wanting to compare the weight changes of several clients need another measure.

Several exist (LeBow, 1981). Of them, one that appears quite useful, albeit difficult for clients and therapists to initially attach meaning to, is Feinstein's (1959) reduction index. It evaluates actual loss in relation to required loss—loss needed to attain ideal weight (Wilson, 1978). It does so by multiplying the proportion of overweight lost by the proportion of overweight at time 1. Percentages are then obtained by multiplying the result by 100.

$$\text{Reduction index} = \frac{\text{pounds lost}}{\text{pounds overweight}} \times \frac{\text{weight at time 1}}{\text{ideal weight}}$$

Another informative measure, already discussed in chapter 1, is Quetelet's body mass index. Decreased body mass would be equivalent to body mass at time 1 minus it later on. Using more than one weight measure is desirable, and weekly progress is best reflected by absolute weights.

Charting Weight Progress

Box 4.1 is used to follow each client weekly. Linear and metric heights and pre–post BMIs are written down on the chart, as are three weight statistics: initial goal, best weight (including BMI), and desired loss. To illustrate this form's yield, consider a fictitious client named Martin Klin. Let's say he's a 38-year-old married factory worker with three children, each of whom is under 13 years of age. Also let's say he's been in treatment several months for debilitating anxiety experienced at work and home, and now, having prospered, asks for help with a weight problem.

Standing 6 ft 2 in., he begins this phase of his treatment at 240 lbs. These statistics are written on the upper portion of the table. His initial goal for sixteen weeks (the interval could be longer) is 220 lbs. That's a 20-lb loss from the beginning, roughly 1.2 lbs weekly and is an acceptable rate of loss.[2] Sixteen weeks is sufficient to make a first step. To lose

---

[2]Ideally a baseline could follow this initial charting. It would be used to gather pre-treatment information on the client's nutrition and weight.

Box 4.1. Weight Progress

Client's Name: _____ Martin Klin _____ Age: 38 Sex: M

Height in inches: 74 Height in centimeters: 188

Weight:		Pounds	Kilograms	BMI
Pre-treatment		240	109	30.9
Initial Goal for 16 weeks		220	100	
Best Weight		180	82	23.2
Desired Loss		60	27	7.7

	Date m/day	Weight	No Change/ Loss/Gain	Amount Change (for week)	Cumulative Loss
Starting	1/8	240	nc	—	—
Ending Wk.	1 1/15	238	L	2	2
(Circle	2 1/22	236	L	2	4
weight	3 1/29	237	G	1	3
data	4 2/5	235	L	2	5
recorded)	5 2/12	236	G	1	4
are in	6 2/19	234	L	2	6
	7 2/26	233	L	1	7
_____	8 3/5	231	L	2	9
pounds or	9 3/12	230	L	1	10
kilograms	10 3/19	228	L	2	12
	11 3/26	228	nc	0	12
	12 4/2	226	L	2	14
	13 4/9	224	L	2	16
	14 4/16	223	L	1	17
	15 4/23	222	L	1	18
	16 4/30	220	L	2	20
			BMI Post-treatment		28.3

substantially, however, Mr. K. will, of course, require more time. After four months, a follow-through contract would become operative, and sessions would become more intermittent.

Next best weight and the difference between it and the starting weight are listed. The result is the overall desired loss. Set with both published standards and client preferences in mind, best weight is for him an ideal. For Mr. K., it could very well be set at 180 lbs. It would be arrived at by asking him about what he feels a good weight for him is and by assessing where on the 1983 Metropolitan weight tables in appendix 1 he's placed. (Controversy over whether to use the 1959 tables of desirable weight or the newer 1983 tables exists [Simopoulos, 1986]. The newer charts are more lenient, especially among those of short stature—desirable weights are 12 lbs heavier for men and 14 lbs heavier for women [NIH, 1985].)

I've included the 1983 norms in appendix 1. Guidelines for using them are as follows:

1. With the client in light indoor clothing, without shoes, measure height.
2. Add one inch before reading across the table because it was standardized on individuals wearing one inch heel shoes.
3. Look in the medium frame-size category, unless you have accurate information on the client's frame-size.
4. Take the mean of the two numbers in the category.

No clear information on Mr. K's frame-size is available; therefore, we consulted the chart according to a medium-frame man and found that he should weigh 175 lbs. That's below his own estimate of best weight— 180 lbs. Whatever the compromise, it's important for the stipulated best weight not to loom as an impossible hurdle. If initially best weight is set high, new weight goals can be revised downward as old ones are reached.

When graphed, the grid of the table of Mr. K's week to week changes would be jagged. Note the grid contains five pieces of information: session date, session weight (specified in pounds or kilograms), direction of session change (no change, loss, gain), amount of change from the last session, and cumulative change. Thus on January 29, Mr. K. weighed 237 lbs, a gain from the previous session—he put on 1 lb and by so doing brought his cumulative change to 3 lbs. If as part of treatment, therapist and client negotiate a reinforcement for weight loss clause in a broader body-shape change contract, the last column of the table, cumulative loss, would determine when reinforcers would be forthcoming. It is this column that tells if change from basal weight (the client's lowest recorded weight) has occurred.

Elements of charting weight extend beyond working a scale and keeping a record. Clients may be uneasy about being weighed or chagrined over failing to progress and say:

I had a bad week, loads of violations. Wish I could just forget about last week and start again. I know you'll be disappointed in me.

In return, the therapist could say:

We all have bad weeks. I would rather have you learn why yours was lousy than to forget about it. You can always start over, but it's best to find out about your mistakes before you do. And don't worry about me being disappointed in you, I won't be.

The weight check prompts the therapist to explore the client's past week and uncover how lost weight was in fact lost. That some clients resort to unhealthful stratagems to reduce has been mentioned earlier. It was pointed out that contracts focusing on weight loss but excluding behavior and energy changes may, for some, promote taking laxatives and relying on other dubious mechanisms for reducing.

I started this section mentioning that for clients and therapists alike, weight loss is a favorite marker of progress. It is clear, simple, readable, reliable and meaningful. Yet as the only barometer of a program's effectiveness it is wanting. As just said, it may reflect the outcome of some insidious pattern the client has adopted. It alone tells you little about the client's behavior modifications. And it is not, upon reflection, the major goal. Becoming thinner, more than becoming lighter, is the real hope.

TRACKING SIZES

In the units they're measured, sizes change slower than weight does. Therefore, in this program, sizes—circumferences and skinfolds—are tracked less often than weekly. Monthly, as box 4.2 indicates, is sufficient. The top third of this table would portray the client's waist, chest (bust), arm, hip, and thigh measurements. It also would disclose the waist–hip ratio (see chapter 1). For some clients, tracking size differences is exhilarating. They'll eagerly welcome the chance to try on clothes they've outgrown and with nearly equal gusto visit shops to see if they can now fit into smaller garments. I remember one young man I treated who enjoyed spending part of his Saturdays downtown at a local department store trying on pants. As he managed over the weeks to squeeze into waist sizes closer to those he identified as befitting his peers, his customarily somber mood brightened.

Others remain incredulous, seeing no reason to explore and find out if there's been any of this sort of progress. A client might inform:

Client: I know I've lost weight, but I'm still as fat as ever. Now I believe what you said awhile ago about weight and fat being different.
Therapist: You're right, they're not identical. But remember I also said that weight loss and fat loss usually do go hand in hand over time. Let's look at your progress record (show circumferences and so on, if there's been

Box 4.2. Circumferences, Skinfolds, Calories													
Circumferences*	S**	1	2	3	4	5	6	7	8	9	10	11	12
Waist													
Hips													
Waist/Hip													
Chest (Bust)													
Upper Arm													
Thigh (R or L)													
Skinfolds (mm)													
Triceps													
Biceps													
Suprailiac													
Subscapular													
Calories													
Daily Recommendation													
Average Daily Actual													
Wealth***													

Circumferences* are in (Circle): inches, centimeters
S** = Start of Program. Numbers following it are month intervals.
Wealth*** Derived from pounds times 3500 calories or kilograms times 7700 calories.

a positive change). You've gone down in your waist and chest, more so in the waist. This means that you have had a recordable improvement in the way clothes now fit you.

Readily available size-change data can attenuate the motivational decline that happens when clients feel that the process of losing weight is cumbersome and the actual loss slight. A drop in waist size, for instance, is concrete proof of a program's effectiveness, justifying to the client the efforts taken. Like weight change, it is powerful and meaningful.

Not as easy to interpret, however, either for client or therapist, is the next class of information box 4.2 reveals, namely skinfold data—triceps, biceps, suprailiac, and subscapular. By measuring such sites, as disclosed in the first chapter, one is attempting to determine the level of subcutaneous fat and generalize from it to total body fat. Though controversy about such a fat assessment exists, taking skinfolds represents yet another convenient way for the practitioner to mark the client's body-changes from time 1 to some later moment in therapy.

Clients are told:

It's helpful to track fatness changes by not only seeing your sizes alter, but also by pinching you with this device (caliper shown). It doesn't hurt. It estimates fat.

Mostly I'm interested in if what I'll measure changes over time. I'm going to measure the right side[3] of you each time, and I'm going to mark the exact place I want to measure with this pen. Ok? Also, so I can be surer of what the true measurement is, I plan to measure you more than once right now, and I'll do that every time I measure you, too. Do you have any questions?

More specific information could be added, based upon the Grimes and Franzini (1977) guidelines considered below, about measurement sites and client requirements. These guidelines are for the four skinfold sites named in box 4.2. By summing results after measurement, one can estimate the client's percentage of weight composed of fat. Published standards are available (see Durnin & Womersley, 1974).

Guidelines for Gauging Skinfolds

1. *Triceps site:* taken over the midpoint of the muscle belly, midway between the olecranon (elbow) and the tip of the acromion (the highest point of the shoulder), with the upper arm hanging vertically (Edwards, Hammond, Healy, Tanner, & Whitehouse, 1955). Note: if the examiner suspects that the triceps muscle has been pinched up with the fatfold, the subject should stiffen the arm (to define the muscle) and then relax it for the measurement. The mid-point of this site should be measured and marked with a felt pen, since subcutaneous fat varies considerably in this area.

2. *Biceps site:* marked and taken over the midpoint of the muscle belly with the arm resting. Note: since the examiner is measuring from the client's side, care should be taken to locate the midline of the biceps. This is easier if the subject is seated with the back of the hand resting supinated (palm up) on the thigh.

3. *Suprailiac site:* taken 3–5 cm above the iliac-crest (tip of the top of the hip bone) in the midauxillary line (a line dropping from the armpit as if along a shirt side seam). Note: loosen any tight-fitting garment (e.g., belt) covering this area several minutes before taking this measurement. Also with the extremely obese client, the examiner may need to push gently through the layers of adipose tissue to locate the crest of the iliac.

4. *Subscapular site:* taken 3–5 cm on a line from the inferior angle (bottom tip) of the scapula (the flat triangular bone in the back of the shoulder) at an angle of about 45 degrees to the vertical with the patient's shoulder and arm relaxed. Seltzer and Mayer (1965) suggest that this skin-fold be taken "in a line slightly inclined in the natural cleavage of the skin." In this area subcutaneous fat is ordinarily rather uniformly distributed. Note: for women, the bra back-strap may cover this site and should be unhooked several minutes ahead of time to allow any adipose tissue compressed out of that region to return.[4]

---

[3]Researchers differ on side of the body from which skinfolds are taken. Durnin and Womersley (1974), however, find no major effect resulting from side of body.

[4]From W. B. Grimes and L. R. Franzini, Skinfold measurement techniques for estimating percentage of body fat. *Journal of Behaviour Therapy and Experimental Psychiatry*, 1977, *8*, 65–69. Reprinted with permission of Pergamon Press.

The assessor needs a caliper (e.g., Lange or Harpenden) capable of exerting $10g/mm^2$ (Seltzer & Mayer, 1965) at the site of measurement. Reliability, more so than validity, is of most importance to the practitioner. Sites are frequently reduced from four to one; triceps is the easiest to gauge, and the Grimes and Franzini guidelines for doing so are useful. Also useful is the compatible and now classic advice that Seltzer and Mayer (1965) offer:

> The skinfold measurement to be obtained is the (doubled) thickness of the pinched "folded" skin plus the attached subcutaneous adipose tissue. The person making the measurement pinches up a full fold of skin and subcutaneous tissue with the thumb and forefinger of his left hand at a distance of about 1 cm from the site at which the calipers are to be placed, pulling the fold away from the underlying muscle. The fold is pinched up firmly and held while the measurement is being taken. The calipers are applied to the fold about 1 cm below the fingers, so that the pressure on the fold at the point measured is exerted by the faces of the caliper and not by the fingers. The handle of the caliper is released to permit the full force of the caliper arm pressure, and the dial is read to the nearest 0.5 mm. Caliper application should be made at least twice for stable readings. If the folds are extremely thick, dial readings should be made three seconds after applying the caliper pressure.[5]

TRACKING OTHER BODY VARIABLES

Mentioned before were blood lipids, such as low density and high density lipoprotein cholesterol, as well as blood pressure (diastolic and systolic). With consultation from a physician, they and other barometers of physical health can be tracked during treatment.

---

[5]From C. C. Seltzer and J. Mayer (1965). A simple criterion of obesity. *Post Graduate Medicine 38*, 2, August p. A-104. Reprinted with permission.

Five

Tailoring a Treatment and Involving the Client: Energy Variables

TRACKING NUTRITION

Adequate functioning requires macronutrients of carbohydrate, fat, and protein and micronutrients of fat soluble vitamins A, D, E, K, water soluble vitamins B and C, and minerals (e.g., Iron, Calcium). Moreover, there must be a continuing source of water.

Carbohydrate supplies energy. The monosaccharides, simple sugars (glucose), are a main source, fueling the central nervous system. Though depleted quickly, glucose is stored as glycogen. Protein also supplies energy. Protein is a complex combination of molecules comprising amino acids that repairs and builds tissues. The body synthesizes all but eight of the 22 amino acids; these eight are the essential amino acids and are supplied only through the diet. Without them, the reparative and constructive functions of protein cannot take place. Fat (saturated, monosaturated, polyunsaturated) is the largest energy source capable of storage for long periods by the body. For moderate and light physical activity, it is chiefly fat that empowers. Moreover, it is fat that is rich in vitamins to preserve healthy skin. Only one fatty acid, linoleic acid, cannot be synthesized. Although having no energy value, water is required for the body's chemical reactions. Vitamins and minerals also must be present (Carroll et al., 1976).

Because dieting so easily leads to deficiencies in the forenamed macronutrients and micronutrients, tracking nutrition, especially while the client restricts intake, is advantageous. Tracking the nutritional quality of the client's diet requires a standard for comparing the data after each check. Most accepted is the Recommended Dietary Allowances (RDA). These guidelines (see appendix 3), determined in part empirically and in part judgmentally, are recommendations for healthy populations. Individuals suffering from specific conditions are not considered. What's more, the RDA guidelines are not written with dieting persons in mind. Indeed, the RDAs may well be different for those restricting intake and markedly increasing activity.

Dietitians are likely to be the best-trained professionals to make both routine and special (for the client with special needs) nutritional assessments. There are computer programs for profiling dietaries and a comparatively quick (seven minute) checking procedure that uses three-day diet records (The Nutrition Company, 1984). The practitioner can augment the nutritional level of diets by urging the client to look for nutritional bargains—foods high in nutrients for the calories they yield—and to partake of a varied diet, one that samples from the food groups of meat and fish, breads and cereals, dairy products, and fruits and vegetables (see Epstein, Wing, & Valoski, 1985).

TRACKING CALORIES

Albeit fundamental in dieting, calories per se are not identical with nutrition. Granted, certain numbers of calories form the base around good nutrition, but no number guarantees that nutrition is good. In fact, the obese high-calorie-intaker may be malnourished and feel sluggish (Deutsch, 1976). It's not the high number of calories that's preventing the nutrition from being good, it's the dietary constituents.

As has been indicated, calories (meaning kilocalories) are units of heat, energy for life-sustaining processes and muscular work. An imbalance of calories means calorie intake and calorie outgo are unequal. When intake exceeds outgo, the inequality, if protracted, produces a gain in fat.

Tracking Intake

Tracking calories is more difficult than tracking weight and size. Reliable and valid records of calorie intake are hard to come by (Lansky & Brownell, 1982; Zegman, 1984). Yet, obtaining accurate calorie counts, which necessitates accurate measurement by clients of what they eat and accurate conversion of these measurements into the energy units of calories, is fundamental. Unfortunately I can offer no sure-fire way to get high quality data, only six helpful steps (see also Zegman & Baker, 1983).

Teach the Client to Value Calorie Counting. Some clients are experts when it comes to knowing the amounts of calories in foods even though they are unable to make the knowledge work for themselves, whereas others come into treatment uninformed. For both groups, I find indicating something close to the following helpful:

> Let me say a few words about calories. Calories are not *in* foods per se. We often talk as if we consume them, but we don't really. We eat food with energy that under the right conditions serves us. Calories is a convenient term to measure and compare and evaluate. In this program counting them is important. The information you get helps in making decisions.
>
> For one thing, by thinking in terms of calories, you can compare foods. For example, what's the difference between eating an apple or having a slice of apple pie? The apple has 100 calories, the piece of apple pie 410 calories. You may want the pie, regardless. In order to plan meals carefully, however, it's vital when choosing the pie to know it's 300+ calories more than the apple. Knowledge of calories is valuable for the dieter because it adds information to decisions about what to eat.
>
> It's also valuable for the exerciser. We'll discuss exercise more fully later, but for now let me point out that just as with foods, you also can compare the calories of activities. For instance, what's the best way to pass the time between 4:00 and 4:30 this afternoon? If you sit it out, you'll spend about 1.3 calories a minute. If you instead take a walk, you'll raise that rate to about 5 calories a minute.
>
> What's more, calories can be a bridge between food and activity (Konoshi [1973] provides a cornucopia of illustrations). Suppose after eating that apple pie, you want to exercise it off. That amounts to figuring out the numbers of calories the pie brings to you and then determining how active to get. If walking burns about five calories a minute, then a piece of pie with its 410 calories is worth a lot of walking. But figuring this way is inexact, because even if you did nothing in the realm of physical activity you still would be expending calories—remember just living burns up a lot. Nonetheless, use calories to compare foods with activities. The advantage is realizing that expending energy helps counterbalance consuming it.

Teach the Client to Calorie Count. Because more manageable tasks are more likely to be done, demonstrate weighing and sizing food portions. Have clients try to do this and give them feedback. Food models are useful in training (e.g., Nasco Life/Form Food Replicas, Modesto, CA 95352). Seeing the difference between the traditional 100 gm serving and the typical home serving is illuminating for numbers of clients.

Furthermore, point out the difficulty of calorie-costing dishes that contain a combination of foods (e.g., casseroles). Recommend, when it is impossible to weigh separate ingredients, estimating amounts of the ingredients and multiplying the guess by 1.2—adding 20%.

Make an Effort to Liberalize the Daily Intake. The goal of therapy is fostering at least a 1–2 lb weekly reduction. Drastically lowering intake, as some clients swear you must do to get weight off, may cause such problems as failing to comply with treatment recommendations. Surely, a client getting solace from food may find the lowering, if severe, intolerable and do almost anything to escape it. By increasing exercise opportunities while decreasing intake, the practitioner engineers a therapeutic energy equation that places less of a burden on the calorie intake term. Liberalizing the diet improves cooperation.

Suggest Calorie Counting Simplifications. To make calorie counting easier, advise clients to put favorite dishes on 3×5 cards. Even better, when possible, is have them type daily menus on personal computers and access the information as needed.

Give Proof That the Calorie Records Are Important. Practitioners who postpone checking clients' food records risk receiving sloppily kept data, or perhaps no data at all. A good practice, as said before, is to back up the calorie monitoring assignment by scrutinizing, in the clients' presence, their recorded attempts at doing it.

Enlist a Helper. Lastly (although this list is not exhaustive) have someone periodically observe what the client eats during several meals. Records can be compared later. All disagreements (e.g., foods, amounts, calories) should be discussed. Of course, as has been indicated, the client must agree in advance to the person selected as observer and to the practice of being observed. Helpers, as disclosed, may be spouses, children, other family members, or friends.

Obtaining a week's worth of daily intake records requires not only a willing client and a data retrieval device (see box 6.2) but also a daily calorie intake allotment. This calorie assignment will vary along with clients' needs, practices, weights, ages, sexes (RDA, 1980). Considering 3500 calories the energy equivalent of 1 lb of stored fat—7700 calories the equivalent of 1 kg of stored fat—the loss of the 1 lb is equivalent to a 3500-calorie deficit. By this logic, a daily deficit of 500 calories will result in a weekly loss of 3500 calories—1 lb (.454 kg) of fat. That the hope embedded in the calculation does not often become a reality is one of the great disappointments faced by weight control therapists and their clients, alike.

Some practitioners, having insufficient data to make a cut of 500 or 1000 calories or simply preferring published diets, will recommend an established low-calorie bill of fare. Others will employ an exchange system, which allows choices within food groups and results in a set level of daily intake—1200, 1400, 1700 (e.g., Stuart & Davis, 1972).

I have clients plan their own diets and collaborate on finding an initially effective calorie intake. Markers of effectiveness are weekly weight losses in the range of 1 lb to 2 lbs, minimal hunger, and few undesired side effects. Quite often the dose for awhile that meets these criteria is seven calories per pound, 15.4 per kilogram. In either system, body weight is multiplied by calories to give the daily intake requirement. Adjustments in the calorie multiplier are made if weight losses go under or over the weekly criteria—raise the calorie intake if losses are excessive, lower it if losses are deficient or absent. But to help from compromising adequate nutrition, keep intakes from going much below 1200 calories a day. (For short, light but nonetheless overweight clients, upgrade calorie expenditure while lowering intake to maintain them at a sufficiently high four-figure calorie intake.)

The bottom third of box 4.2 has space for a year's tracking, month by month, of recommended daily intake, which usually varies little day to day, and also has space for tabulating actual mean daily intake over the month. The client's food record form (box 6.2), when filled out daily, yields the raw data for this last calculation. Because as weight is lost calorie needs for weight maintenance decline, the daily recommended intake requires periodic revision. To illustrate, a 200-lb individual reducing 25 lbs on a sustained program of 1400 daily calories will need less intake, more outgo, or both to continue prospering.

Tracking Wealth and Outgo

Wealth in energy is assessed by finding the product of desired weight loss (box 4.1) and calories, 3500 calories if weight is calculated in pounds and 7700 calories if done in kilograms. Assessing calorie wealth is once again translating weight into energy—the first time we did so was for devising a daily calorie intake. The bottom of box 4.2 provides for making the monthly riches assessment. Though warned of its imprecision, clients are nonetheless told to think of this total as some finite amount of manageable tasks. It is a number that time well spent, not herculean effort, will help erase. Bankruptcy is the goal (Sharkey, 1974).

If the practitioner is successful, the client will begin to expend more calories through activity. Table 6.1, to be detailed in the next chapter, is for tracking the calorie outgo that occurs when therapists bring in exercise as a central obesity control tactic. Activity recommendations, however, may be profitably made earlier during eating control.

I want to be absolutely clear in pointing out that the calorie-arithmetic of weight loss is imprecise. The calories that are spent do not precisely predict the weight that is lost. Nonetheless, by thinking in calorie terms, clients have a useful dimension to evaluate their decisions about foods and exercise.

In this chapter, as in chapter 4, I've begun to clarify what therapists and clients are to do and to discuss piecemeal the treatment package I and my coworkers rely on. In the narrative to follow, I will continue the discussion. Appendix 2 lists session tasks.

Six

Tailoring a Treatment and Involving the Client: Planning and Recording

This chapter continues with the logic of the two previous: in order for practitioner and client to tailor treatment, they must track the obesity triangle's components. We have just discussed body and energy variables. In this and the next chapter our examination turns to behavior. Numerous activities, such as accepting an offer to dine out, watching television, and filling the shopping cart with high-calorie goods qualify as reasonable behavioral targets. But without corroborating data that such actions are in fact the client's difficulties, that's all they are, reasonable targets.

As indicated, this program eschews targeting a priori lists of do's and don'ts (a cover-all-bets philosophy) in favor of looking for specific behaviors characterizing the client (a cover-best-bets philosophy). Tailoring is discovering actions that interfere with and those useful in maintaining a propitious and sufficiently lengthy imbalance of calorie intake to calorie outgo. All interventions that target behaviors for change assume that it is through these changes that desired body differences result. The spirit of this assumption is that targeted actions must be personally relevant to the day-to-day functioning of each client.

There are five classes of behavior for therapist and client to discuss and track that are central to this discovery process: planning, recording, searching for discrepancies between predictions and performances, recouping, and reflecting. The client's role is to self-monitor, self-analyze, and with the therapist examine the data garnered from these actions. Critical therapy topics emanate from this scrutiny. Many clients fail to show difficulties (see Baecke, van Stavaren, & Buremia, 1983) until beginning an obesity reduction program. Therefore, therapists actively need to uncover the client's dieting and exercise difficulties. This is done

by structuring planning and recording tasks. Knowing which of the re-
medial strategies of chapter 2 (e.g., contracting) clients are likely to profit
from awaits discovering these difficulties. Identification precedes
intervention.

As always, the therapist's role in this process is listener, teacher, supporter, collaborator, giver of feedback and praise. In a climate of understanding and trust against a backdrop of rapport, the therapist initiates,
stops momentarily (when client needs demand), and returns to the discovery process.

BEHAVIOR ONE: PLANNING

Plans are forecasts. To plan, one has to organize available or readily
accessible information and then lay out intentions. In this program,
planning is the initial step clients take to bring to light the obstacles,
threats, and dilemmas they face in their daily struggles to reduce.

Planning Meals

Clients are to compare intentions with actions to find violations—that
is, to find how they veer from their own dieting agreements. The first
link in this chain of self-discovery is planning intake.

Box 6.1 is for doing this. If more meals are planned than the four
allowable on this form, more forms are used. Down the first column,
clients list the foods they propose to eat for each meal. On Wednesday
morning, June 8, for instance, an egg, toast with margarine, grapefruit,
and coffee with milk could be listed. Clients would indicate quantities,
calories, and preparations. In the space marked "total" they would write
the sum of all the calories proposed on that day. It would be subtracted
from the daily goal (top right), if less than the daily goal, in order to
tabulate the day's deficit (bottom right). Deciding also to set aside a sum
of calories for unexpected eating—eating that is unplanned—clients
could, next to "slush fund," write 200 calories.

Clients are encouraged to plan meals well ahead of eating. Some have
no difficulty doing so as much as 12 hours ahead, forecasting an entire
day the evening before; others find doing so impossible. Dieters more or
less in charge of preparing their own meals seem to be better able than
their less involved counterparts to plan long ahead. Those tightly controlled by the food requests of family and friends find long-range planning difficult.

I *encourage* planning as much as a day ahead, because within limits,
the longer the interval between intention and action the greater the
chance of food-based problems surfacing. For example, a 5 ft 5 in., 194-lb,
32-year-old woman I have seen for quite some time noted soon after

---

Box 6.1. Meal Plan

Initials: _____ Day & Date _____ Daily Calorie Intake Goal_____

MORNING MEAL

| Food | Quantity | Calories | Preparation |

AFTERNOON MEAL

| Food | Quantity | Calories | Preparation |

EVENING MEAL

| Food | Quantity | Calories | Preparation |

SNACKS

| Food | Quantity | Calories | Preparation |

Slush Fund Calories _____

Total _____

Deficit from goal: _____

---

beginning treatment that when she planned dinner one or two hours before it happened, few, if any, difficulties arose—her actions and plans coincided. But when she planned the dinner menu after breakfasting, she ran into trouble. Her children would frequently upset her intentions with high calorie demands. By long-range planning, she learned cognitively and affectively how closely she was tied to their whims.

Meal planning can be shaped. To lengthen the planning to performing interval, have clients start with a short period (e.g., planning just prior to eating) and then gradually extend it, plan earlier and earlier. Before doing this, test out different times—the evening ahead of the forecasted day, the morning of that day, just after having had an earlier meal (planning lunch after breakfasting). To help those who find planning itself difficult, ask them to start with one meal and then gradually raise the criterion. Sometimes, especially with clients unfamiliar with constructing menus, it is helpful initially to plan meals with them.[6] Later, ask them to get the job done without your assistance. Client perceptions of planning being an odious chore are modifiable, in part, by suggesting that they— as said earlier—use a card file of customary foods or program their home computer with typical menus.

Guidelines to Convey About Meal Planning

1. *Do not exceed the daily calorie objective.* As indicated, daily calories may be set as the product of the client's weight in pounds times seven or eight calories or weight in kilograms times 15–17 calories. The proviso is that the daily intake not become less than about 1200 calories without consulting a physician or dietitian.
2. *Do not undercut the daily calorie objective too much.* A difference over 100 calories is considered too much because it's indicative of poor planning. Giving clients calorie goals that are in round numbers (e.g., 1500) inhibits undercutting for arithmetical reasons. Other reasons, such as feeling that only a low intake leads to weight loss, have to be dealt with in sessions.
3. *Do not try to plan everything to be eaten.* Encourage avoiding inflexibility. Have clients set aside a portion of the day's calories—a slush fund—for unplanned episodes of eating. The slush fund, albeit small, may reduce the feeling that even the slightest violation ruins the diet. Knowing that there are calories available for unplanned eating, no matter if unequal to what's consumed, does help some clients feel that "everything is not lost" if they slip. Indeed, without the slush fund more than just a few clients will turn the minor setback of an unplanned doughnut into the catastrophe of quitting the program altogether. I recommend clients try a 200 calorie slush fund, or about 15% of the day's allotted intake.
4. *Seek the assistance of those close to you.* If feasible, clients with families are to try to involve them in meal planning. The therapist might say: "Find out about your family's foods. Ask for help in planning meals whether or not you're the cook. If you don't, you'll increase the risk that those close to you will complain about your choices . . . and

---

[6]The Auto-Nutritionist III is an IBM or compatible computer program that gives food choices at designated calorie levels. Write N² Computing, 5318 Forest Ridge Road, Silverton, Oregon 97381 for information.

those complaints can be troublesome, causing a planning breakdown. Give your family a say in your meal plans. You'll stand the best chance of gaining their cooperation if you do."

5. *Do not become a diet-food fanatic.* Planning meals of usual foods is preferable to esoteric, "low-cal" goods; stockpiling many diet foods is to be avoided. The therapist could caution: "Be wary of those low-cal foods in special parts of the supermarket. They usually cost a lot and sometimes fail to keep their promises. Read labels. Maybe what's there is just less food."

6. *Look for nutritional bargains.* This caveat of planning asks clients to upgrade gradually the quality of their diets. They are to search for nutritious foods, nutritious for the calories they provide—foods that are part of the compact dietary (Deutsch, 1976). So as to eat the same as other family members do, clients are slowly and progressively to substitute nutritional bargains into the family's customary choices. They are to do so openly, after enlisting the family's agreement. Foods that are high in calories and relatively low in nutrition are not to be forever banished, just regulated.

7. *Try not to plan lopsidedly.* Clients are to avoid the ritual of daytime starving followed by nighttime stuffing. They are to distribute calories throughout their waking hours. Clients are told that perhaps a special meal is planned, so cutting back on other meals is desirable. But such times should be minimized. Lopsided planning is to be the exception.

8. *Do not substitute excessively.* There is a difference between adaptive and nonadaptive replanning. It has to do with the frequency with which plans are modified, and the care with which they are conceived. Changing well-thought-out meal plans once in awhile to recover from unexpected, undesired circumstances differs from doing so frequently and capriciously. Nonadaptive replanning, as opposed to adaptive replanning, results from hasty predictions. To explain the difference, the therapist could tell the client: "Between lunch and dinner, let's say, you eat the last slice of last night's cheesecake, and feel it wise to alter your meal plan for dinner, which you've already constructed— you decide to drop dessert from the menu. That's adaptive replanning. Situations like that don't happen all that often, and you do try to plan meals carefully. On the other hand, let's say you go about meal planning feeling you can easily abandon your proposals. And you do so frequently. That's nonadaptive. What I want you to do is plan with foresight, the foresight you build by learning about yourself."

Planning Activities

Activity plans during the eating control part of treatment are generally just agreements by the client, made in the therapist's presence, to get more exercise. The client may agree to walk or bike daily for twenty minutes and the therapist checks up by asking for a progress report the next session, helping solve problems of sedentariness.

Activity plans made during the activity part of treatment (see appendix 2 and below) are more formal and complex. Aspects of the sessions devoted to it are described next.

Discriminating Activities

The client learns to separate prolonged activities (e.g., jogging, skiing, tennis) from brief ones (e.g., taking stairs instead of elevators, walking less than 15 min.). In other words, sports and recreations are differentiated from daily routines (Brownell & Stunkard, 1980). The brief actions are to be event-recorded (see table 6.1), whereas the prolonged ones are to be calorie-costed.

The impact of brief activities is difficult to measure by counting calories. Brief activities are viewed as beneficial because their positive effects summate. To drive home this point, clients are told:

> Think about these two women. Ms. Smith and Ms. Jones. Both eat about the same number of calories daily, and each is nutrition-conscious. Unlike Ms. Jones, however, Ms. Smith is sedentary. She's not a mover. She would rather drive everywhere than walk anywhere—she's good at finding parking places near store entrances. She rarely goes for the stairs, usually takes elevators and escalators. Her children run up the stairs when they can—child's play, she believes. Instead of mailing her letters herself, she asks her son or daughter to walk the block to the post box. Work-savers fill her home. She has three extension phones and is contemplating another. Her best friend on the block walks to her home four times to every once she reciprocates.
>
> Ms. Jones, like Ms. Smith, plays tennis once a week, but that's about the extent of sports-play for the both of them. Yet Ms. Jones walks to transport herself whenever she can. She does not mind getting things herself and carrying them. She does most of her own errands. She has one telephone and hates the thought of buying another. She often parks her car at the far end of the parking lot to avoid having it bumped and scratched. Stairs don't bother her. She prefers them to stuffy elevators; if she has to go more than four floors she walks part of the way and then takes the elevator.
>
> Even though the same in height and body frame, Ms. Smith is 25 lbs heavier and two dress sizes larger than Ms. Jones.

As for sports and recreations, clients and therapists should be more concerned about duration instead of speed or intensity. Duration is a better dependent variable for evaluating progress. Clients initially may hold that in order for exercise to work, for it really to use up calories, it has to be intense. They may feel that it's only through jogging, or its equivalent, that progress is possible. To them, especially those with recent histories of little or no exercise, the therapist might say:

Jogging (or another intense activity) can be a valuable part of your life, but you have to work up to it. Jogging and other strenuous exercises are not the only ways to burn up calories. As I told you, you're always expending energy—you're doing that just living. Jogging, handball, tennis, racquetball are wonderful ways to *increase* the calorie-burning that goes on, but so are bike riding around the neighborhood and walking. And for you right now these less strenuous exercises are probably better because they're gentler. Did you know that walking an hour is equal in calories to 30 minutes of fairly fast jogging? True, the jogging burns up more energy than the walking does each minute, but the walking lasts longer—twice as long. Time counterbalances speed. So, when you finish exercising you don't have to be out of breath for it to have done you some good.

Selling the Active Life

Advantages and perceived difficulties of the active life—some repeats of previous discussions—are frequently addressed at this stage. These tenets are included:

1. It preserves and protects lean body mass (Oscai, 1973).
2. It may increase post-exercise metabolic rate (Thompson, Jarvie, Lahey, & Cureton, 1982).
3. It may attenuate a diet-induced drop in metabolic rate (Donahoe, Lin, Kirschenbaum, & Keesey, 1984; Stern, 1984).
4. It results in cumulative calorie losses.
5. It is self-correcting (Mayer, 1968).
6. It may attenuate appetite (Epstein, Masek, & Marshall, 1978; Mayer, Roy, & Mitra, 1956).
7. It makes dieting less severe.

Objections commonly voiced by clients include hating it, finding it publicly embarrassing, worrying that it will just increase hunger, worrying that doing it may be physically harmful, worrying that to pay off it must be herculean.

Typically dialogue at this point in treatment is as follows:

Therapist: How do you feel about getting more active?

Client: Won't it be too stressful for me? After all, it's been years since I've really exercised.

Therapist: I don't mean just exercise but also the briefer daily routines I talked about. As for exercise, if you go slowly it won't harm you. Your physician has said that there is no reason for you not to do it. What you must remember is be prudent. Stop if there's any pain. Take it easy.

Client: Well I don't mind taking out the garbage and things like that, but I hate the thought of really exercising. I'd rather just diet.

Therapist: You're not alone. Many people would rather diet. They loathe exercise. But it can help you in ways dieting can't do alone. For one thing, exercise does something extra towards getting you thinner. It minimizes losses of that part of you, the lean you, that you don't want to reduce, while it brings about changes in fatness—that part you do want to reduce. Research shows that people can lose a goodly amount of fat without losing much weight at all.[7] It also shows that some can lose the same amount of weight but widely different amounts of fat and lean tissue. One researcher,[8] for instance, treated about 30 overweight women by having some diet, some exercise, and some do both. Those who dieted ate 500 less calories a day. Those who exercised expended 500 more a day. And those who did both, dieted and exercised every day, ate 250 less and expended 250 extra. So, in terms of calorie imbalance, each group was equal, that is 500 calories a day was dropped out, either through having people eat less, move more, or do both. After 16 weeks, weight losses were totaled, and on average each person lost about 11 lbs, no matter which of the three treatments they had had. But when fat losses and changes in lean tissue were measured those who had exercised or who had dieted and exercised to lose, compared with those who had only dieted, lost 35% more fat. Those who had just dieted not only had lost less fat they had also lost the most amount of lean tissue, something they certainly didn't want to have happen.

There's another thing about exercise. It takes a lot of the burden off dieting. Recall, to lose you have to expend more calories than you consume. Raising your expenditure of calories by exercising means that you don't have to lower your consumption as much by dieting. What I'm saying is that you can bring about a calorie deficit that pays off for you by eating less each day, moving more each day or, best of all, doing both.

Another thing, if you exercise regularly and build up slowly, you'll probably get physically fit. By that I mean you'll improve stamina, lung efficiency, heart work at rest and at play, and the ability to take in and use oxygen. Many physical things will get better.

And for yet another thing, if you're regularly active and you happen to gain a little weight—let's say you go on vacation—exercise will help take you back to where you were before you gained.

Furthermore, exercise has been known at times, after you finish a bout of it, to shift your metabolic rate upwards. You remember the metabolic rate discussion. Suppose you hit a plateau. As I mentioned, sometimes to adjust to fewer calories when dieting, the body gets more efficient and responds by needing fewer calories. And you know what happens then: it's harder to continue losing. There's evidence that exercise helps lessen that kind of efficiency. As I said, it may be the only way you have of dealing with those plateaus.

Client: Yeah, okay, but won't I just eat more if I exercise?

Therapist: Not necessarily. In fact, a little bit of exercise may curb the appe-

---

[7] Johnson, Mastropaolo, and Wharton (1972) subjected 32 female students to a 2½ month program of physical conditioning and found that for the 20 completers body fat decreased significantly but not weight.

[8] Zuti (1972). For details and examples of this finding see also Dressendorfer (1975); Oscai (1973); Zuti and Golding (1983).

tite. When I go to the gym at noon, I want less food, if I do eat immediately afterwards. Walking briskly may do the same for you. Try it out. Many years ago a well-known nutritionist, Dr. Jean Mayer, found that of the people he studied those engaging in a light amount of activity ate less than those remaining sedentary. He looked at quantity of food eaten and amount of work accomplished in about 200 Bengalese jute workers. Hard workers were big eaters, as you might expect, but so were those who didn't move around all that much.

Client: Even if exercise is as wonderful as you say, wouldn't I really have to do a tremendous amount of it to lose weight? I'd really have to walk to lose a pound, wouldn't I?

Therapist: Yes you would. But don't think of exercise that way. Don't think of trying to walk to lose a pound all at once. Just think of enjoying a mile's walk, spending about a 100 calories of your calorie wealth, your riches. And think of enjoying it every day for a month. In that amount of time you'll have used the calories in that pound and had a good time, too. Too slow? Well, just fix on this: if strolling daily were to have been your routine for, let's say, the last five years, the calories in about 50 pounds of fat would have been burned up. That doesn't mean you'd be 50 pounds lighter. But the calorie benefits of exercise do accumulate. You have to be patient.

Client: You're probably right. I can't wait for things to work. But there's something else. I don't want anyone to see me exercising.

Therapist: Why do you say that?

Client: It's obvious, isn't it? How can I dress for exercise and leave the house like this? Might as well hang a sign on my back that says "look at the giant slug."

Therapist: Is that how you think of yourself—as a slug?

Client: Well, not now, but when I exercise I'm sure I look funny.

Therapist: I hear what you're saying. But I want you to think of exercise as medicine to take in order to feel better. Would you continue to take it if the sight of you doing so displeased others?

Client: Of course I would. But that's different. Taking medicine is quick, and nobody laughs at a sick person.

Therapist: Why don't they laugh?

Client: Because sick people can't help being sick.

Therapist: I think what you're telling me is you deserve being laughed at because you feel you're at fault for being fat.

Client: Yes, I guess I do feel that way. I'm weak.

Therapist: It's not weakness that's fattening. It's a lot of other things. We've discussed many of the knowns and some of the unknowns about obesity, and weakness is not in either category. Right now, you're trying to do something that takes lots of responsibility—being here and working hard.

Client: Yes, this program's no fun.

Therapist: Okay! I'm suggesting another part that's no fun, at least right now. Today, it's medicine. Tomorrow, I hope it's pleasure. For now take the medicine, and don't let insensitive and uncaring people tie you in knots, preventing you from something you need. You have as much right as anyone to exercise. You have to exercise your rights and your body. If you won't walk fast outside in shorts, wear slacks and walk slowly. As you become more active, reservations about being active in public will lessen. Move more and chances are you'll want to move more.

For clients still wanting to know more about activity, I'll suggest readings (e.g., Sharkey, 1974, 1984).

The Activity Plan

Teaching to plan activities is teaching to use table 6.1. Clients are told to plan brief and prolonged activities for each week. The brief, as said, are event-recorded and the prolonged calorie-costed. Some plans involve new changes and others repeats of old changes.

To explain, consider the new changes portion of the table (bottom part) first. On it, let's say, the client states such brief activity intentions as climbing stairs at work Monday, taking out the garbage at home Tuesday, and walking briefly (about 10 min) to get the evening newspaper at the corner market every night; one or more activities may be planned to happen on several days. Likewise, let's suppose, he or she states such prolonged activity intentions as riding the bike 30 min Monday evening, walking around the park 20 min Wednesday, walking around the park 40 min Friday, and swimming 45 min Saturday. Not only is duration forecasted but also calories expended. Appendix 6 gives rates for computing total calories.

But the calorie data are imprecise. Calorie expenditure tables fail to indicate the net increase in calories used by doing the exercise. Garrow (1976) points out that net value, value to the client, is the calorie cost of whatever else the client would be doing instead of exercising subtracted from what the exercise yields. Also, calorie tables are based upon a 150 lb standard body weight. Heavier clients will expend more than lighter clients when doing the activity—about 10% more for each 15 lbs above this standard. Conversely, lighter clients will expend about 10% fewer calories for each 15 lbs they are under the standard (Sharkey, 1974). Weight of client, in other words, alters the exercise's worth. (Appendix 7 shows clients this phenomenon by providing an algorithm for setting calorie expenditures that reflects weight changes.) Furthermore, the tables are imprecise because they fail to consider fitness differences. Someone in superior condition who raises pulse rate to 130 bpm by exercising uses more calories than someone in poor shape who manages the same feat. The conditioned person, however, must do much more than the unconditioned individual to raise pulse rate to that high level (Sharkey, 1974).

Regardless of these interpretive problems, clients are encouraged to mark progress and set objectives in terms of calories expended. They are to do so because this is a most useful barometer for tracking activity. Calories expended is a dimension that for many clients increases in meaningfulness as weight losses ensue. Put differently, clients can see

Table 6.1. Activities: Old and New

Week of _____

Past Changes to Be Repeated

	Monday	Tuesday	Wednesday	Thursday	Friday	Saturday	Sunday
Brief Activities							
Prolonged Activities	Plans CE Goal	Plans CE Goal	Plans CE Goal	Plans CE Goal	Plans CE Goal	Plans CE Goal	Plans CE Goal

Past Changes CE Goal = _____   New Changes

	Monday	Tuesday	Wednesday	Thursday	Friday	Saturday	Sunday
Brief Activities							
Prolonged Activities	Plans CE Goal	Plans CE Goal	Plans CE Goal	Plans CE Goal	Plans CE Goal	Plans CE Goal	Plans CE Goal

New Changes CE Goal = _____

Total CE Goal For The Week = _____   Total Violation Calories For The Week = _____
Total Violations in Brief Activities = _____   Total Violation Calories Recouped = _____

the accumulated benefits of being active vis-à-vis being sedentary by tracking the calories that they spend—avoid saving. And from this review, they can then consider the gain of weight that they have helped prevent. If eventually encouraged by the signs of progress their efforts generate (e.g., a certain level of calorie outgo weekly), they will be more likely to continue being active.

Consider now the "past changes . . . " half of the table (top). In this portion, the client is to plan to repeat activity triumphs, brief and prolonged, of the past week, endeavoring to make total and partial successes cumulative. The focus is on last week's accomplishments, not promises. Only triumphs are targeted for repetition. Let's say, for instance, that during the week of May 8, the client finishes 20 minutes of the planned 40-minute Friday walk, expending 150 calories. For the week of May 15, the table would have to include, on the past changes half for prolonged activities, this 150 calories.

It need not all come from walking and it need not be planned for Friday, but it must total to 150 calories of activity. Clients are permitted to substitute freely in order to vary their activity lives. As for brief activity repeats, they are likewise to target last week's successes; with the brief events, however, they are to try to reproduce these accomplishments on, when possible, the previously stipulated days.

The initial plan is predicated on data from the interview and session discussions. After this first week of planning activities—the week when only new changes are forecasted—the entire form is completed during each meeting. That is, clients are to propose new changes and the repetition of past ones in the therapist's presence. When carrying out plans, they can combine the new and past change proposals—walk 30 minutes on Saturday to fulfill a planned 20-minute new change and a 10-minute past change for this day.

With therapist functioning as collaborator and supporter of gradual upward shifts in activity, the client constructs the coming week's plans; past, new, and total calorie expenditure (CE) goals are filled in. The objective is building a comfortable regimen of daily routines and exercises. Within two months of the start of this process, clients will be doing a dozen or so brief activities (to be increased over time) and expending through exercise between 900 and 1000 calories weekly (see American College of Sports Medicine, 1978).

BEHAVIOR TWO: RECORDING PERFORMANCE

Both planning and recording involve monitoring, but they differ in what's observed: planning tracks intentions—intentions to eat, intentions to be active—whereas recording looks at actual happenings. Planning is pre-behavior monitoring; recording is post-behavior monitoring.

The accuracy of records is often an issue. I stress to clients that it is only by knowing what *does* happen that there's a chance to affect what *will* happen. Estimating accuracy by assessing reliability is possible as said by asking significant others to be periodic checkers. For example, a spouse may write down foods consumed and exercises completed by the client for two of every fifteen program days. Percent agreement rates would then be tabulated. Clients usually know they're being observed—unobtrusive reliability estimates are nearly impossible—and so may well be uncharacteristically accurate on these check-up days.

Meal Recording

Completing meal records, as in box 6.2, requires clients to document each of their day's episodes of eating. Immediately after finishing a meal or snack, they are to complete one of these forms. For example, suppose four meals are planned. The client would make a record on a meal record form as soon as one of them or an unplanned repast is finished. The letters at the top, BLDS, stand for breakfast, lunch, dinner, snack, which is followed by meal number to that point in the day. Down the columns is space for type of food eaten, quantity, calories, and preparation, and below each box is room to total calories. The chart keeps the observer informed about what's been eaten and the calories accumulated up to then—calories up to the meal and including it. The last line is for totaling the day's calories. Also, there's space to note when a meal begins, feelings prior to, during, or following it, and remarks.

Activity Recording

Recording activity is much simpler. All clients have to do is make a check mark underneath the planned activity on table 6.1 when they complete it. If they fail to live up to plans, however, the recording task becomes more involved. They have to first mark a *V* for violation underneath the planned activity and then, elsewhere (as will soon be discussed), write out the particulars of why they violated plans.

Making the recording of inactivity—failing to carry out plans—harder than the recording of activity is like punishing behavior that needs weakening and rewarding behavior that needs strengthening. Self-monitoring may weaken behaviors that result in it and strengthen ones that avoid it because self-monitoring soon becomes dull and boring, even though it alerts and astonishes clients about their unwholesome living patterns. I'm not saying that recording successes is unrewarding, rather that tabulating data becomes tedious.

The growing aversiveness of self-monitoring doesn't work against the

---

Box 6.2. Meal Record

Initials: _____   Day & Date _____   Daily Calorie Intake Goal _____

Meal   B   L   D   S   # thus far today _____
              Type   Quantity   Calories   Preparation

Food 1 _____

Food 2 _____

Food 3 _____

Food 4 _____

Food 5 _____

Food 6 _____

Food 7 _____

Food 8 _____

Total Calories for Meal _____

Time Begin Eating: _____

Feeling: _____

_____

Remarks: _____

_____

_____

_____

TOTAL CALORIES THUS FAR TODAY _____

goal of diminishing unwanted eating—indeed, refusing a snack to avoid having to record it is helpful. But self-monitoring would be contra-therapeutic and work against the goal of increasing activity if inactivity was ever chosen over it to avoid having to record the activity. One way around the dilemma of making the unpleasant act of recording contingent on a behavior to be strengthened, namely activity, is to not design the contingency at all, meaning that clients would not have to self-monitor. Yet failing to take data and thereby prevent written feedback about progress would also be contra-therapeutic. The alternative, done here, is to make being active easier to record than being inactive. The client has to *write* about plans not followed.

Graphing

There are two graphs, one described here and one described in chapter 8, that over the course of therapy clients are taught to make and vigilantly keep up to date.

The Initial Goal and Best Weight Graph. This is a simple line graph portraying the correspondence of weight in pounds or kilograms on the ordinate to weeks during training and follow-through on the abscissa. In addition, two other horizontal lines of different colors are drawn, one being the initial weight goal and the other (lower down) the best weight (see box 4.1). Clients are to post this graph, for instance in the kitchen, and mark it weekly.

The next chapter illustrates yet other records that clients are instructed to make.

Seven

Tailoring a Treatment and Involving the Client: Violating Plans, Recouping, and Reflecting

BEHAVIOR THREE: SEARCHING FOR VIOLATIONS

In this program a violation is failing to keep a plan. Violations are discrepancies between eating plans and eating performances or between activity plans and activity performances. Such disagreements may show up as specific food violations—eating an unplanned slice of cheescake. They may be excesses of planned foods—eating twice as much hamburger on the planned sandwich. Less disastrously, they may be eating planned foods in planned amounts prepared in unplanned ways—frying potatoes instead of mashing them. They may show up as noncompliance with brief activities—failing to take the stairs at work, or be deficiencies in carrying out prolonged activities—walking only 20 minutes of the forecasted 40-minute walk. There are various ways violations may appear.

Information about them gives therapists the targets for intervention. Clients gather the information and therapists, joining them, review and analyze it, as well as devise remediative strategies. This work is an alternative, in the wake of self-recrimination, to turning the setback that is the violation into the catastrophe of stopping all efforts to reduce. As one client writes:

> I know I must dedicate myself to this task and not feel totally defeated when or if I slip. This has been my pattern in the past, and I need to alter it. Anything worthwhile takes time—remind myself of this every day.

In a climate of understanding and acceptance, clients report difficulties in following plans and their self-discoveries. They are asked to search for and record in their diaries three main parts of each violation: particulars, substance (including feelings, before, during, and after), and theme(s).

Particulars and Substance of the Violation

As for particulars, clients are to write the time, day, and date of the violation and what number for the day it is. If the violation is food-based, clients also should note how many calories are acquired from it, which equals the calories in the extra minus those remaining in the slush fund. Thus, eating 300 calories worth of unplanned cookies and having 150 calories left in the day's slush fund makes the calories acquired from the violation 150. If, instead, the violation is activity-based—involves exercising—clients are to determine unspent calories. Forty-five minutes of swimming instead of the planned hour amounts to a 15-minute violation; the calories in the 15-minute lapse would be tabulated and logged in the diary.

After enumerating particulars, clients are to write about the violation itself, detailing what happened. A client states:

> I walked into the house after work tired and angry and ate cashews, which were a gift. There must have been two pounds. I hate cashews, but I just didn't want to stop. I'm sure I ate a pound at least. Once I was buried in the cashews my mood really became horrible. I was angry, depressed, aggravated and feeling awful because of the salt. Afterwards, I felt like a pig, really as if I have no willpower.

When possible, clients should indeed document feelings before the violation (tired and angry), during it (hating cashews but not wanting to stop, increasing anger, and so on) and afterwards (feeling weak-willed). Writing about feelings is instructive. Clients are encouraged to put them down on paper, even those independent of a specific violation, and later review them during sessions.

A depressed client in her sixth week of therapy writes:

> I have had another rough week. I didn't even keep track of what I ate. I did a mental count though. I wanted to be down in pounds today, but I don't think I will be. I am depressed in spite of my efforts to fight it. I'm sorry I did not try harder. I know it's me who's going to suffer if I don't get this weight off. Is this babble making any sense? I have trouble concentrating. My thoughts wander and I forget what I'm saying in the middle of it. I really don't think I could remember what I ate two days ago, unless I wrote it down. I've got to try to not be so hard on myself and just accept things the way they are.

Themes of the Violation

Each violation has one or more, often interrelated, themes underlying it. Particular themes and combinations appear and reappear, describing the intimate challenges clients face while struggling to reduce. Violation themes tell about the *whys* of plan violations, the reasons blocking progress. Clients are to write down the themes they see.

Eating-Plan Violation Themes

A comparison of plans and performances (box 6.1 and box 6.2) could reveal such violations as an unplanned doughnut in the afternoon and unplanned dinner in the evening. These would be noted on box 6.2 by placing the letter *V* beside the times they occurred. When thinking about the first violation, the client might make the following diary entry:

> Left work early with Jim. He promised me a ride home. Nice that he offered, but why did he have to push that doughnut on me? He said he bought several at lunch and didn't finish them—he's a beanpole. "One won't hurt," he pressed. I couldn't say no. He's such a nice guy. It's sure easy to blow the slush fund this way.

For the next violation the client might write:

> Got that call from Clare at Redmonds Jewelers. They said they just received the old Rolex watch I've been wanting. Price is fantastic, way below what I'd thought. Called Jan at work and suggested we celebrate. She asked about my diet, but I pointed out how rare getting a Rolex is. We went to Carbonnes. Enjoyed the Fettucini Alfredo, Antipasto, and Chianti.

The main themes underlying these two violations, to be named in the diary, are in turn *food-friend* and *food-reward*. Food-friends are food-pushers whose kindnesses can cause dieters trouble. Food-friends usually are not evildoers with preconceived goals of stopping one from dieting; they instead, by their actions, say that food and friendship go hand in hand. Food-friends may be coworkers or members of the client's family. A spouse who brings home calorie-laden treats qualifies, as does a parent who prepares an elaborate take-home basket of foods after serving a sumptuous dinner. Food-reward, the second of the themes, is almost a redundancy. Food is so much a part of the pleasanter side of things that many of us, probably most of us, punctuate our good moods with it. We treat ourselves with it after some display of good conduct or good fortune.

Other themes are described below.

Food-Available. This source of violating has to do with the omnipresence of food. Some clients report that because their homes are veritable storehouses of ready-to-eat snacks, they find it difficult to follow plans to avoid snacks. One woman I know, attempting to explain a plan violation involving cookies, related: "Cookies called out to me." She knew where they were and found this knowledge overpowering. Similarly, a 240-lb man I treated reported:

> Came home from work really starving. Began cooking a steak, but couldn't wait. Grabbed for the cheese, large hunk of it, that I knew was in the icebox.

Yet another client, a woman whose husband was her food-friend, pointed out how he created the situation of food availability that she found so bothersome:

> I asked him to buy one bag of jelly beans so I could have some, and he comes home with five bags! I could have killed him! They are too tempting for me, even when I put them away. I hate Halloween because it means snacking on all the things I save for the kids.

Lastly, a client who travels frequently wrote that when the food is included in his room charge—the American Plan—he overeats:

> Was in Banff four days ago. Stayed at the art school up there. They have cafeteria-style eating, really good. They give you meal tickets, and you can eat as much as you like. Charges for the lodging include meals, regardless of how much or often you eat. I ate huge lunches there, even though I never do at home. Just couldn't pass up the opportunity.

Food Presence. Like food availability, food presence, whether alone or combined with other themes, underlies many violations. Also traceable to the omnipresence of food, it however has an added component, salience: those who violate their eating plans do so because they see available food, smell it, or both. Clients reporting that snacking at home on candy is problematic also often report proximity to well-stocked living room and dining room candy dishes. (I know someone who keeps visible stockpiles of candy in the bathroom.)

Food presence is a common source of violating plans. Clients mentioning difficulties controlling their eating at parties find the arrays of food they see there irresistible. For many, the sight of food is indeed a powerful stimulus. Some clients in fact acknowledge feeling sated but nonetheless compelled to eat if they lay eyes on available food. They often report, in addition, that food deprivation can be a critical antecedent of the food-presence situation:

> It was about 6:30 in the evening and I just walked in the house. I was really hungry, because I was too busy to eat lunch. I ate the first thing I saw when I opened the icebox . . . Quiche. Saw some crackers on the counter, ate them too. Then had supper at 8:00 p.m.

Food Conserved. The philosophy of "waste not, want not" leads many parents daily to reprimand their children for leaving food. These mothers and fathers often serve way too much, cajoling their youngsters to eat beyond need. If they fail to make their children comply, they may consume the leftovers themselves and thereby, or perhaps by eating the remains from the serving dishes, violate their food plans. In either case, they are exhibiting a food-conserved problem.

Food Tasting. Clients who cook usually have an initial advantage in planning because they know about recipes and foods in general. But they may be at a disadvantage in following plans if they, as many good cooks do, repeatedly taste each concoction created. Tasting brings in calories and so is to be estimated. The slush fund may be insufficient to handle these extras.

Food Cravings. Many clients say cravings are critical in causing unwanted eating. Food cravings are irrepressible, intrusive, and intense. To exemplify, I'm now treating a woman who reports incessantly thinking about all kinds of meats. Another I'm caring for is bothered, with equal intensity and frequency, by ice cream. Illustrating the tie that food cravings can have with other thoughts and emotions, one woman states:

> My mind is always on sweet tasting food! I would rather forget that food existed, but I know I *eat less when* [client's emphasis] I plan well, at least the scales are showing it. Tonight I'm tired and my son just spilled my [sugar substitute] all over the table. That upset me . . . the mess, and I'm too tired to clean it up. I yelled at him too! I immediately reverted back to my old ways and downed cake. (I went over my limit.) I should have reached for a fruit but I craved something sweet.

Food Outing. When dining out—at a restaurant or friend's or if living in a school dorm—clients' choices of foods are restricted. There's little control over the menu. Food presence may contribute to violating the plan, but the main theme is food outing. Clients regularly forced to eat away from home, particularly those traveling extensively, rarely are able to plan effectively. They rarely know the menus where they dine, and so must calorie-plan. That is, they must forecast the calories they'll allow themselves at each meal, estimate how many they'll take in, and search for the involvement of other violation themes.

Others Eating. When in the company of others who are eating, it is difficult for clients to turn away from foods. A rather short, 178-lb woman in her sixth week of treatment witnessed herself violating her plan because of this social theme:

> Was out with Morna and Kathy at the Craft show. Afterwards we went for a treat. They ordered chocolate cake. Follow the leader syndrome, except that I had apple pie a la mode. Should have had fruit instead. But couldn't bring myself to.

Time Available. Behind this violation is the theme of enduring time by eating. The client, perhaps while waiting for a bus, buys a candy bar at a nearby drug store or, having a few minutes to kill before the next appointment, enters a coffee shop or bakery and buys something to eat. A 213-lb man in treatment writes:

> Three days ago I went down to (discount sporting-goods store in Winnipeg) to buy that new reel I told you about. The clerk said their other store had it, as they were sold out. Promised me he'd have them send it over in less than an hour. I said I'd wait, because going home and back would take a lot longer. Looked around the store for about 10 min, and then grew restless. Thought I'd just go have a cup of coffee to pass the time but while there (coffee shop) just couldn't resist the cheesecake. Still had 15 min to wait after the first cup.

Food Heroics. Those adopting perfectionistic standards (see chapter 2; Mahoney & Mahoney, 1976) easily fall victim to the food-heroics theme. When, in other words, clients repeatedly deny themselves because they believe that only by doing so will they lose weight, they set themselves up for a food-heroics violation. As is rewarding good fortune with food, food heroics is rewarding past denial of food with food. A client writes:

> Got up early and felt hungry. Last night had planned cantaloupe and cornflakes for today's breakfast. Still proud of myself for resisting cherry pie at dinner that everyone else had had, took a slice this morning. Pie was right there on the counter. Told myself it was just the slice I didn't have last night.

This violation involves the themes of heroics and presence. Often the most apt description comes from combining themes. For instance, those whose diets are thwarted on airplane trips are usually victims of an amalgam of food-friends, others-eating, and time-available themes. They are captives of flight attendants, who with little or no provocation provide them and everyone else with food and drink.

The eating violation themes, identified again in appendix 8, are not exhaustive of all possibilities, as the following complex violation—laced with feelings of recrimination and failure—shows. The reporter is an unhappy 190-lb woman.

> I was making kids and husband dinner, preparing it in A.M. so wouldn't have to do it later. Put it on too long, and burned half of it. I was upset—this rarely happens! Their dinner was ruined. I then ate the part that was still good . . . about six pieces of steak. (I wanted to destroy the evidence.) Anyway I then wasn't hungry for lunch. I didn't weigh the steak but it was about 8 oz. But what I did, due to frustration, is nibble on the chocolate covered raisins in the cupboard. Don't know how many I consumed. Too angry at myself to count them. My husband finished them at my request, so I wouldn't. They (husband and kids) had hot dogs. I had fish. My husband said dinner was O.K. But I couldn't accept my failure so I wanted to fail some more by eating the chocolate raisins. Got on the scale Wed. morning and am not down.

The client calls this a food-distress violation. It's that as well as one in which food presence and food availability intertwine with feelings of self-recrimination. Nonetheless, her description is to her more personal and illustrative of the problems she feels she faces. Clients naming other, "non-standard," violation themes in their records, especially those repeated in different settings or otherwise surrounded by different particulars, should not be forced to conform to my listing. They should feel free to write about their violations in the way they view them.

Activity Plan Violation Themes

As said, when clients fail to live up to activity plans they mark their charts (table 6.1) with the letter *V*. Not only are brief activities sometimes violated but so also are prolonged ones, either partly or wholly, and themes may occur singly or in combination. Reasons for violating are as follows:

Activity Excessive. Too much too soon is planned. The problem occurs especially among those overweight men and women who have been regular exercisers in the past. The theme involves confusing past accomplishments with current hurdles. Clients committing the activity-excessive violation forget that time and the accretion of fat weaken one. I recall a fellow I saw who, to renew his lost affection for exercise, proposed to swim 40 minutes three times during the week and run six miles seven times. I couldn't dissuade him. Years ago, he had run as much as 10 miles in one mini-marathon, but since then had been fairly inactive. By the second day of his new herculean regimen, he quit. In his words, "It wiped me right out."

Too Unimportant for Activity. Clients at times report being unable to fulfill their activity plans because another individual has used up the time they had set aside for exercise. The other individual is usually a friend who visits or calls *about nothing in particular*. The client has difficulty being assertive enough to say, "Let's talk later, I have to go."

Activity Visible. I've already commented on the aversion many of the overweight have about being seen exercising. It is rooted in our appearance-conscious, thin-crazed society that says the fat should hide. Indeed many individuals, numbers of them themselves obese, act as if the fat should turn invisible. Dressing for exercise is particularly difficult, because few exercise garments were ever designed with the overweight in mind.

Too Busy for Activity. Therapists encouraging clients to become more active frequently encounter this resistance, "I don't have time." Clients may well not have time because of bad scheduling. Time management is needed. Sometimes, though, the problem is letting an unexpected event intrude upon planned activity. One client remarks:

> Was about to go downstairs and ride the bike (stationary bike). Don (husband) called about the taxes. He reminded me that I promised to gather all the receipts. I guess I didn't have to right then, but I just felt I had to get it over with. Used up the activity time—Alan (son) and his friends came home after school as usual.

This woman's violation is categorized as too-busy-for-activity. She allowed a postponable task to intrude upon a planned exercise. She felt an urgency to complete a task that could have waited and because of this, or rather because she succumbed to the urge, lost an opportunity to be active.

Forgetting About Rainy Days. There are reasons the original activity plan has to be set aside. The theme here has to do with lacking alternative exercises, times, and places when the unavoidable happens. Reasons for plan changes occur that (unlike being too busy for activity) are uncontrollable, such as encountering bad weather or having to care for your ill child.

Activity Is Boring. Some clients have difficulty choosing prolonged activities. They feel few exist and find it hard to vary their activity lives. This contributes to growing tired of exercising. Therapists have to show that there is more to being active than jogging or swimming and that exercise need not be a solitary affair.

The Activity Sparer. There is at least one theme that underlies brief activity violations. It involves others who discourage the client's becoming more active. The activity sparer insists that the client take the least effortful route. Also, like the food-friend, the activity sparer is kind and out of kindness that's hard to refuse does seemingly nice things or sees to it that they are done. The nice things deprive the client of the chance to be active. An activity sparer may be a spouse who, instead of having the client walk to the corner for the newspaper, arranges for home delivery. Or the activity sparer may do all the chores around the home rather than delegate any of them. Or the activity sparer may be a coworker who insists on giving the client a ride rather than permit walking, or who is uneasy about some felt potential dire consequence of activity (e.g., "Better not walk to the mailbox, it's freezing and you'll catch cold").

Appendix 8 lists themes both of eating violations and activity violations. Clients are given the listing to help them learn to track their plan violations. Discussion, rehearsal, and feedback occur in sessions.

BEHAVIOR FOUR: RECOUPING

Recouping minimizes violations and lessens the catastrophic implications of a setback. As noted, turning the setback of a minor violation of the dieting or exercise commitment into the catastrophe of quitting weight reduction efforts entirely, by continuing to eat excessively or by stopping exercise altogether, or by doing both, is all too common among clients. The distortion in thinking that accompanies this pattern is probably something like, "I'm just too weak-willed to stick this out, so why bother trying."

In addition to having slush funds for their food violations and staying free of rigid dieting and exercising standards, clients are to examine ways to attenuate the effects of plan violations. They might, for instance, divide excess calories obtained from unplanned eating or failing to exercise as forecasted by the remaining days of the week and then, using the calorie reduction figure they derive, take in less and expend more each day until the violation is recouped. Recouping tries to neutralize the violation's effects, both calorie and cognitive, and (to repeat) tries to prevent minor infractions from blowing up into major disasters.

Clients are to attempt to recoup if the planned calorie expenditure is unattained or when the day's calorie allotment is exceeded—the slush fund makes recouping some food violations unnecessary because it covers them. Clients are cautioned against meal skipping as a way to recoup from food violations. For example, when writing of a food plan violation involving food availability and feelings of frustration over being "housebound," a woman in her eighth treatment week notes: " . . . so to compensate for the extra calories, I missed lunch, and then my mood was really horrible (anger)."

She also reported doing a fair amount of exercise after skipping lunch to "burn off" calories—however, her response to doing so was even more anger, because her unfortunate choice of activity was floor-scrubbing. Clients are warned not to attempt to overcome violations through major bouts of unpleasant work.

Moreover, leaving the recouping of exercise violations that occur during the week to the weekend, a frequent practice, is discouraged. The best recouping strategy is, for the next few meals after the violation, calculating a specified reduction of calories and stipulating a reasonable number and duration of "makeup" exercises.

BEHAVIOR FIVE: REFLECTING

Clients are now asked to consider ways to stop breaking plans, and to write their ideas in diaries for discussion in therapy. By exploring themes of past violations, they are more likely to tune in to impending violations and, as a result, develop better, achievable plans. They are to analyze themes contributing to recurrent and infrequent violations, both of which produce extra calories or which prevent their dissipation. And they are to suggest ways of dealing with these themes. This type of reflecting, making specific reflections, is analogous to Mahoney and Mahoney's (1976) fourth step, examining alternative solutions to problems, except here the targets are obstacles interfering with keeping agreements with oneself.

Another type of reflecting in which clients are encouraged is *general reflecting*. General reflections are about one's special relationship to food and activity. Also, they are about renewing the weight-loss commitment, as this client's words indicate:

> I want to be allowed to start over again, a clean slate as of today. I have just had this week to re-think my priorities and realize that I am no good to myself or anyone else the way I feel. It is time I took charge of myself and my life. I will make a daily schedule and write down an exercise time each day and I will do my homework re: what I am eating. I have allowed so much to get in the way of what you are trying to help me accomplish that I have practically gained back all the weight I lost! This can no longer go on!!! I am not looking forward to the summer because of the way I look and feel. No one else can do this for me. It's up to me but I need more time to do this. Will you help me? I have felt scared that I only had 16 weeks to achieve a goal and instead of letting it work positively—I knew I couldn't achieve what I wanted in that time frame, so I think I was acting in a self-defeating way. I must no longer think like this. It is not healthy. I will adopt the idea of one week at a time, one pound at a time!

She did start over. She was disabused of thinking she had only 16 weeks to succeed—there's no time limit. If she wished, she could renew contracts and take vacations from the program.

Another client, also introspective, writes:

> My violations are most definitely food availability, food presence, food craving and, to a small degree, food tasting if I'm doing a lot of cooking. *Food craving* is the most serious violation—I will think of food and seem to have to have it. My problem is with my relationship to food and not my outside world but rather the me inside. No one or nothing in my environment is making me think of food or compelling me to eat.
>
> My worst lack of control occurs before my period—I crave sweets, salt, bread. I seem to lack the strength or discipline to continue to eat the foods which I know will make me feel better and help me lose weight. I have difficulty getting through a day according to plan. What does this say about my personality? Maybe the answer to my problem is not food itself, but I feel it's a habit like biting nails. Is it that I should learn something or am I missing something in my personality? Is there something I do or feel that will not allow me to lose weight? If it affects my life by making me unhappy, why do I continue to eat so much?
>
> Sometimes I feel I want to burst out of myself—I would like to find a way to interrupt my eating. There are times when I feel light and empty and although I weigh 200 and more pounds, I still feel good. However, I can't seem to hang on to that empty feeling. Maybe if I could understand what I lack I could handle the problem. Do I lack control?

Several therapy sessions were devoted to this reflection. Her notion that it's what's inside—her personality—that is the trouble was identified. Addressing her statement "No one or nothing in my environment is making me think of food or compelling me to eat," my colleagues helped her explore her external environment and the ways it might incorporate her feelings and thoughts. The importance of affect and cognitions was kept in the forefront as she came to see how food deprivation during the day affected her wanting to eat, and how the presence and availability of some foods caused her anguish.

The related issue of control was in part externalized by helping her find tasks to battle feelings of helplessness. Eventually she did such things as eat regularly and buy vegetables to munch on instead of starving throughout the day. Control was not left as an undefined, invisible personal attribute.

Her naming of food cravings as a problematic theme—she named it here as well as in a few of her specific reflections—was also addressed. After reviewing her proposals for dealing with it, her therapist (my supervisee) and she agreed to try to put 15 minutes between the urge and its fulfillment. During the interval she was to think about the desire and read a list of prepared and personally relevant reasons why she did not have to have the urge-foods. This worked well for her sometimes.

Another partially successful strategy was simply including a few of these foods into her plan, thereby removing the allure she attached to them and the disastrous psychological effects of giving into temptation. Although it wasn't tried, she could also have been directed to plan how many of the urge-foods she would buy and gradually, over time, reduce their number. What's more, she could have listed pleasant alternatives to eating, acting on them when the compulsion to eat struck (see Stuart, 1978a).

There are various ways to modify the themes of violations—sometimes, as indicated, simply identifying them is salutary. Specific reflections are the client's first thoughts on what to do. During sessions, the therapist, collaborating with the client, should attempt to find out how recurrent particular themes are and help develop feasible and tailored solutions. For instance, naming an others-eating violation, a client explains:

> I had several of these this week, as I wrote. Three happened at work. Two more involved social eating with friends while out after my aerobics class. Mary and Betty wanted to go for cake after class. They ordered it and it seemed hard to resist. I didn't resist the urging from others who were also 'grazing.' Felt deprived.

Her first reflection was: "Take along low-calorie snacks." Then, she thought: "I should have knitted that sweater that is in progress. I took it with me just for that purpose—to knit while others ate—but didn't do it."

During the session, her records and reflections were reviewed. Others-eating violations were frequent that week, and before it as well. Knitting the sweater while others ate was abandoned for two reasons: it already hadn't worked in one of the settings, and it didn't even attempt to include the perception of deprivation. Taking along lo-cal snacks was acceptable to her for dealing with others-eating problems at work, but was seen as awkward for those encountered at restaurants with friends— there, to her, it was just too noticeable. Consequently, she decided to include modest desserts in her food plans for the days she wasn't at work but expected to have others-eating violations. She *intended* to order desserts at coffee shops when accompanied by her friends. The strategy worked well.

Designing tailored approaches to handling violation themes is a collaborative effort. Thus, following discussion, one might use assertive responding to deal with food-friend violations, after practicing, through imagery techniques, saying no to food-friends.

Assertive responding could also figure into a client's exercise violations. Let's say failing to walk the full number of minutes planned is due to someone—a well-meaning associate perhaps—frequently or even occasionally interrupting plans. Or if the client misses out on exercising because unforeseen but postponable tasks seem to intrude, he or she might invoke stimulus-control technology to better manage time. (Stimulus control also seems particularly well-suited to food availability, food presence, and food conservation themes.)

Contracting could be useful in food-reward situations by having the client substitute more propitious outcomes for memorable occasions. It might also figure prominently in reducing the boredom of activity—perhaps by incorporating monetary payoffs for compliance or by increasing the reliability and performance of an activity partner (e.g., LeBow, in press).

The techniques of chapter 2 may be applied in various combinations to deal with various violation themes. The eventual product will be controlled largely by the obstacle the client demonstrates and what is agreed upon to remedy it.

Eight
Following Through

Now comes a most difficult and critical part of therapy—following through. For the client, following through means trying to continue or maintain progress. Follow-through contacts should be part of the overall treatment plan (see chapter 3). For numbers of the overweight and their therapists, continuance and maintenance are the heartaches of the process of trying to manage weight, for it is during them that hard-won progress may stop and relapses begin. Present-day technology—nutritional, psychological, psychiatric, physiological—gives no sure-fire methods to forestall these disasters. But there are worthwhile and practical suggestions to offer. To be clear, continuance is when the client, not yet having reached best weight (box 4.1), strives to do so. Maintenance follows continuance. Or possibly maintenance interrupts continuance, relieving it, if the client decides to stop for awhile at a weight that's heavier than best weight, trying not to backslide.

CONTINUANCE

A significant part of therapy is helping clients establish and re-establish effective ways to work toward best weight. The end of the first phase, training, occurs when the client reaches the "initial goal" (box 4.1) and feels comfortable doing the program. It marks the start of the second phase, continuance, which for most is necessary because best weight has not as yet been achieved.

Ingredients of a Potentially Successful Continuance

Continued Contact with Therapist. Clients are given a listing of points to remember (table 8.1) about treatment and instructed to refer to this list often. They continue seeing the therapist intermittently until reaching best weight, either the original proposed or some newly negotiated

Table 8.1. Points to Remember

Overall Points
1. Strive to eat a balanced diet.
2. When choosing foods, look for nutritional bargains.
3. Distribute your calories throughout the day.
4. Enlist your family's cooperation when making dietary changes and when planning meals.
5. Watch for feelings that would let the inevitable setback (e.g., eating some high-calorie treat or failing to exercise as hoped) become a catastrophe. **Call the therapist when you have these feelings.**
6. When your recreational life is varied, combine past and new exercise changes.
7. Keep to a schedule of exercise in which you expend between 900 and 1000 calories a week.
8. Strive to develop an active, comfortable regimen of daily routines.
9. Check and mark your weight graph weekly.
10. Check calorie wealth weekly.
11. Check sizes monthly.

When trying to reduce
12. Set a calorie-intake level that's approximately your present weight times seven or eight, so long as you stay very near 1200 calories per day.
13. Make an intake plan daily that has a slush-fund.
14. Make an activity plan weekly for brief and prolonged activities.
15. Record adherence to both types of plan each day.
16. Search for plan violations daily.
17. Record plan violations as soon as possible after committing them. Pay attention to their particulars and especially their themes.
18. Recoup gradually from violations.
19. Reflect upon violating plans and attempt solutions.
20. Contact the weight control therapist when you feel violations are getting out of hand.
21. Attempt to garner support and help from family and friends.

Other Points*

---

*These are points that are specific to the client being treated.

one. How intermittent contact becomes varies from once in two weeks or three to monthly or to every two months. The speed of fading contact is collaboratively determined, progress toward reaching best weight being a main datum. Planned telephone checks may be part of continuance but are no substitute for face-to-face meetings.

Continuing Program Steps. Clients are to go on using the problem-solving tactics (e.g., searching for themes of their violations), employing a schedule that they set and modify. For some, this means daily planning, recording, and so on, for a while. For others, it means rapidly arriving at a periodic schedule. Clients are told that continuance is self-determined. They are to set their own timetable for doing the program. We do, however, recommend a gradual process that is *paced with continued progress*—perhaps daily to twice weekly to once weekly to once every two weeks. Clients are informed that even one week a month on the program helps them track violations.

They are encouraged to explore various schedules, such as two days in a row out of every ten or twenty. It could also be that during the continuance phase, as indicated, clients vacation from the program. Perhaps they grow weary of it; perhaps they actually do go on a holiday and don't want to plan, record, and so forth; perhaps they find themselves in a stressful situation and want to stop procedures. Whatever, the temporary objective becomes maintenance. And it is useful at these times to reinforce the decision to maintain rather than continue losing. Clients are told that it is unrealistic to try to reduce during vacations because new and different foods and unfamiliar surroundings are likely to prevent them from doing so. Better to enjoy the holiday than fail and feel badly. Job changes, sudden increases in work, and family crises are all likewise among the worst times to persevere in attempting to reduce.

When not doing program steps, clients are to try to follow such weight reduction policies as looking for nutritional bargains, keeping to a reduced daily calorie allotment, and exercising, but are to neither plan nor record their efforts. The program is arduous and time-consuming and usually our clients welcome this break, so long as progress is not unduly thwarted. Another advantage of reducing the written-monitoring chore is creating the chance for just mentally tracking behaviors, a practice consonant with the exigencies of the post-treatment environment.

Checking and Marking the Weight Loss Graph. Vigilance is crucial. Clients have to know the effects of their efforts in trying to attain best weight. Therefore, they are to register weekly weight on the best weight graph (see chapter 6). Daily weight checks are discouraged. When weighing for graphing, clients should dress in light indoor attire and keep the week-to-week times for weighing similar.

Marking Size Changes. At training's end, clients are reminded of the size changes that have occurred to date (see box 4.2). They are to continue to check, track monthly, and record these data in their diaries; also, they are encouraged to track the fit of clothes. Some clients, experiencing slow weight losses and an inabillity to "see" their own progress, relate how friends, especially those they only get together with now and then, remark on their "looking thinner." Only a record of propitious size changes will corroborate these satisfying and motivating social validity data.

Hazards of Continuance

In addition to following the recommendations, clients in the continuance phase are also made wary of several of its interrelated potential hazards.

Allowing the Scale to Rule Mood. As just implied and mentioned much earlier, weighing frequently is undesirable because doing so may give false feedback that creates a self-fulfilling prophecy. That is, the dieter witnesses a meaningless upward shift that generates unhappiness, guilt, lowered self-esteem, less self-control and owing to all this, eventual gaining. The therapist might say:

> Remember, as we discussed weeks ago, resist being the sort of person who leaps upon the scale every 24 hours or more often. Don't let that bathroom scale shape your day's mood, for if you do you may needlessly worry about a gain that's not fat, undergo an anguish that's undeserved, and worst of all, let yourself feel so badly that you do badly.
>
> You know, your scale can show a gain that has nothing to do with getting fatter or failing to get thinner. For one thing, the scale may be off. For another, you may be retaining water . . . meaning you're heavier, not fatter. Women may see this monthly in concert with their menstrual cycles. Carbohydrate lovers, both men and women alike, may see it as they express affection for pastries, cookies, and jams, even though their caloric intakes are moderate. So may those fortunate enough to have their food worlds under control and their exercise lives in full swing, for when fat is shed water is produced. What I mean by that is simply that water is produced from the process of burning up fat, and as a result, weight is not automatically lost as soon as fat is lost. The water has to go, too, which it soon will, before the scale shows the reduction.

Drifting Accuracy. This hazard of continuance means starting and persisting to err in measuring the calories in foods as well as those expended through exercise. The therapist might warn:

> Look out for drifting accuracy. When drifts happen errors in counting calories arise . . . and they mount up. These errors can be major reasons why your progress toward best weight slows down or stops altogether.
>
> One drift is beginning to weigh food incorrectly. As you know, there are three things that affect the numbers of calories in foods—type of food, preparation of food, weight of food (amount). You may have no difficulty telling one food from another or recognizing preparation differences, but still be easily deceived by quantity. Can you tell by sight alone how many calories are in 200 gm of mashed potato compared with 300 gm of it? If you can't, then when you have the larger serving of potato you may think you're taking in a little under 200 calories when the right figure is closer to 300 calories. With the naked eye it's hard to see the difference. So continue to weigh food while on your way to best weight. To minimize drifts in accuracy, make the scale readings carefully—quick readings often are wrong. Also, periodically compare your records with those of a family member or friend. Track down the reasons for any discrepancies.
>
> As you become more and more familiar with the foods you customarily eat, try first to just estimate their calories, checking your guesses by weighing the foods afterwards. Then, when you prove yourself to be a good estimator, only weigh foods some of the time.

Foods you never think of weighing create problems, too. Is the same sized apple still what you'd call small? What's the difference between a little piece and an average-size piece of cake? Do you still call the peanut butter on your sandwich 66 calories, even though you've switched from a knife to a tablespoon for scooping? Get to know how you define a serving now, and see what others say.

There's another drift to watch for. That's thinking you're expending more calories than you are. Actually, the upshot of this drift is the same as the one before: an unwanted surplus of calories. Check to see if you're still expending those 1000 calories a week. Remember, as you lose weight the number of them the exercise uses up diminishes.

Turning a Setback into a Catastrophe. This phenomenon, one that many of the overweight could without too much trouble say is partly responsible for the starting–stopping scenario of their repeated attempts at weight management (and one named in this book), may occur during training, continuance, or maintenance. A client slips, and, because of the "failure" and its psychological sequelae, quits.

The worst problem is not the slip. It's the reaction to the slip. As indicated in chapter 2, Marlatt and Gordon's (1980, 1984) relapse-prevention training has been adapted to treating the obese (Perri et al., 1984) with some success. We have likewise, over the years, found it desirable to have clients trying to attain best weight identify and rehearse coping with risky slip-generating situations. Equally as valuable is having them also identify and rehearse coping with their affective and cognitive responses to failure. Techniques of discussion, imagery rehearsal, and in vivo practice are applied.

These three hazards may by themselves or in combination cause a decline in motivation to continue striving for best weight. Starting continuance with gusto and the feeling that finally a sensible stand against obesity has been taken, clients may after a few bad weeks lose their enthusiasm. They may begin feeling that the program costs too much in work and time for what it yields. Waning motivation signals premature termination. As indicated, clients are at such times to contact the therapist. Ensuing sessions would focus on feelings, cognitions, and uncovering manipulable obstacles. Among the tactics recommended might be taking a temporary vacation from the program or writing short-term contracts that reinforce compliance with what the client sees as problematic aspects of continuance.

MAINTENANCE

Continuance is striving for best weight. Maintenance is striving to keep it or, if the client stops at an earlier point, keeping to that earlier point. It seems that after undergoing training and continuance or just training alone, keeping to a weight should be easier than is reducing—allowable calories increase, control over eating and activity improves—but unfortunately maintaining after losing is difficult. Indeed, maintenance is a most perilous time, a time when many clients have their hopes and successes crushed.

Before going further in discussing this problem phase, let's distinguish several of its meanings. If weight and fat variables (point A on the obesity triangle) are the major consideration, effective maintenance is minimal or no regaining after training. Lost weight and fat stay lost.

If body components as well as energy intake and expenditure variables are considered (points A and C), effective maintenance is striking a lasting balance between the energy terms and finding that weight and fatness fluctuate little.

If behavior variables (point B) are the top consideration, effective maintenance means that clients continue to apply what is to them useful technology. Compliance does not erode. Also, setbacks trigger renewed efforts to control. In a few words, the client does what's needed to meet the emergency.

Rarely is there reliable evidence of behavior maintenance. Therapists and clients usually look for weight stability. Some therapists, however, do act as if they believe that behavior maintenance is the route to favorable body changes, that weight and fat losses follow designated behavior changes. To wit, clients are sometimes asked what they have done to avoid relapsing. Nonetheless, as noted, the data about the course of this behavioral form or any of the other types of maintenance is scanty.

Though particulars differ somewhat, continuance recommendations are maintenance recommendations, too. Likewise, the hazards of continuance are also the hazards of maintenance. Destructive moods are intensified by allowing the scale too much power, errors in calorie-counting are repeated as client accuracy wanes, and setbacks (e.g., gaining a bit of weight) may turn into catastrophes (e.g., regaining all lost weight and more).

Though not inevitable, these occurrences are threats that often become realities. As yet, there are no guaranteed ways to block them. We do try to, however. In so doing, we ask clients to do the following:

1. Maintain contact. Three-month and six-month, checkups are requested. Early in treatment, the attempt is made to have the client agree to having them occur. Clients also are to call for an appointment any time difficulties they need help with arise.
2. Reapply problem identification, recouping, and reflection methods. This, likewise, is to be on an as-needed basis—when signs of a relapse appear.

3. Read and re-read the points to remember listing (table 8.1).
4. Remain active.
5. Be wary of and ready for slips and their affective and cognitive by-products.
6. Remember that calories provide a useful dimension for surveying the worlds of food and activity, and remember to re-explore these worlds occasionally.
7. Track weight. Clients are to construct a *range of safety graph* (figure 8.1) after reaching best weight. As is done with the initial goal, best weight graph (chapter 6), weight is placed on the vertical axis and weeks on the horizontal, and two more horizontal lines are drawn. But this time the two extra lines represent the range of safety—the range, frequently eight pounds, within which the client's weight is to stay. For example, if best weight is 140 lbs, the lower line of the safety range would be set at 136 lbs and the upper end of the range at 144 lbs. Falling below the range beneath 136 lbs, is to be followed by eating more fruit, whole grain cereals, breads, and so forth. Rising above the range, a far more likely occurrence, is to signal the need to renew previously successful weight loss principles. Clients are to check their range of safety weekly.
8. Track fat. Clients are to assess sizes monthly.

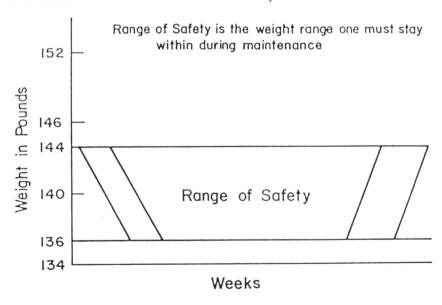

FIGURE 8.1. Stylized graph of maintenance.

We attempt to achieve these objectives through encouraging self-monitoring, having regular checkups (telephone prompts are made), fostering discussion about problems identified and solutions planned and tried, and repeating exhortations to be vigilant and on guard against a false sense of security.

About the last point, clients are told to avoid promising themselves to "take off recently acquired weight this summer" but instead to *do it now*, to reapply the program immediately. Weight, they are informed, changes for several reasons, some unrelated to unwanted behavior patterns, which seems to make program reapplication unwarranted. But one can't be certain if the extra weight is not in fact due to unwanted, remediable actions. So the advice is reapply anyway.

Vigilance is central to stopping complacency. For many, complacency is the biggest problem. Clients are told that they have battled heaviness and fatness during training and continuance and have either won the battle or called a ceasefire. But the war is far from over. It will last a lifetime. They have to guard against being remiss, and must act early enough to interrupt the insidious return of pounds and fat.

Appendix 1:
1983 Metropolitan Height and Weight Tables*

	Men					Women			
Height		**Small Frame**	**Medium Frame**	**Large Frame**	**Height**		**Small Frame**	**Medium Frame**	**Large Frame**
Feet	Inches				Feet	Inches			
5	2	128–134	131–141	138–150	4	10	102–111	109–121	118–131
5	3	130–136	133–143	140–153	4	11	103–113	111–123	120–134
5	4	132–138	135–145	142–156	5	0	104–115	113–126	122–137
5	5	134–140	137–148	144–160	5	1	106–118	115–129	125–140
5	6	136–142	139–151	146–164	5	2	108–121	118–132	128–143
5	7	138–145	142–154	149–168	5	3	111–124	121–135	131–147
5	8	140–148	145–157	152–172	5	4	114–127	124–138	134–151
5	9	142–151	148–160	155–176	5	5	117–130	127–141	137–155
5	10	144–154	151–163	158–180	5	6	120–133	130–144	140–159
5	11	146–157	154–166	161–184	5	7	123–136	133–147	143–163
6	0	149–160	157–170	164–188	5	8	126–139	136–150	146–167
6	1	152–164	160–174	168–192	5	9	129–142	139–153	149–170
6	2	155–168	164–178	172–197	5	10	132–145	142–156	152–173
6	3	158–172	167–182	176–202	5	11	135–148	145–159	155–176
6	4	162–176	171–187	181–207	6	0	138–151	148–162	158–179

Weights at Ages 25–59 Based on Lowest Mortality. Weight in Pounds According to Frame (in indoor clothing weighing 5 lbs., shoes with 1″ heels).

Weights at Ages 25–59 Based on Lowest Mortality. Weight in Pounds According to Frame (in indoor clothing weighing 3 lbs., shoes with 1″ heels).

*1983 Metropolitan Height and Weight Tables for Women and Men. Source of data: 1979 Build Study, Society of Actuaries and Association of Life Insurance Medical Directors of America, 1980. Reprinted by permission of the Metropolitan Life Insurance Company.

Appendix 2:
Program Steps

SESSIONS ONE THROUGH FOUR

- Overview the program (i.e., planning, recording) and arrange for attendance contracts for treatment and follow-through (deposit refund). Obtain a work commitment that stresses client responsibility. A focus on eating may precede one on activity for the first nine or ten sessions. But during the eating control component, activity prescriptions may be profitably given, although the formalized steps of planning, recording, and searching for violations are omitted.
- Where appropriate, state your estimate of success by describing your experience to date.
- Discuss what clients need to purchase.
- Assess the client's social network and interview (appendix 4), letting clients finish it at home.
- Attend to the client's desperation to reduce. Disabuse him or her of the belief that failure in this program confirms that nothing will ever be successful or that it is due to some immutable characterological flaw.
- Explain cycles of weight change and address circumstances that influence week-to-week weight losses (e.g., metabolic rate adaptation).
- Find out about the client's level of physical health, including any dietary and/or exercise proscriptions. Obtain physician input (see appendix 5).
- Begin the tracking of weight, fatness, and calories by starting box 4.1 and box 4.2. Baseline data may follow this initial charting (see chapter 2).
- Explain about the sequence of planning and recording meals.
- Explain about the sequence of finding and recording (in diary) violations. Also explain about the themes of eating violations and how these themes often are combined.
- Explain about recouping and reflecting.

Clients are to adhere to a reduced calorie intake level, first for perhaps two days, next for three days, and then for five days. Each weekly session, therapists are to weigh clients and review records, including diary entries. When not planning or recording, clients are just to try to eat moderately. I recommend shaping program days because it helps reduce feelings of being overwhelmed by the data tracking tasks.

SESSIONS FIVE THROUGH NINE

During these sessions, clients typically have reached seven program days between the weekly meetings. Therapists continue weighing them and reviewing their records at each appointment. Periodic calorie adjustments and size estimations are carried out and graphing is discussed. Special attention is given to analyzing reflections as well as designing remediative strategies and following up on their use.

SESSIONS TEN THROUGH THIRTEEN

Typically now the more formalized activity control portion is begun. And to make the planning, recording, and searching tasks easier for clients, a temporary suspension of food data recording is allowed. As before, weight checks are made each session and size checks more intermittently.

- Discriminate brief from prolonged activities.
- Discuss the advantages of activity.
- Handle objections to becoming more active.
- Explain sequence of activity planning, recording, violation finding, and recouping.
- Explain common themes.
- Explain reflecting.

Program days may be shaped for activity control as they were for eating control, although a full week might be reached sooner—two days, five days, seven days.

SESSIONS FOURTEEN THROUGH SEVENTEEN*

Records are scrutinized as before and suggestions for handling violation themes are checked. During some of these sessions clients are asked to keep both food and activity data.

---

*Typically, after the seventeenth week the follow-through phases of continuance and maintenance begin (see chapter 8). Sessions are intermittent (e.g., biweekly, monthly, bimonthly).

This table is not meant to imply that clients go through the program locked-step. Tasks vary in accordance with client needs. Variations in program structure are common. For example, as indicated, activity prescriptions may accompany the eating control phase. Doing so may well have positive effects on attenuating any diet-induced metabolic rate adaptation. Activity control (sessions 10–17) may be begun before eating control starts, if therapist and client agree that eating problems can wait. A couple may start the program together (e.g., friends). A different shaping procedure, including none at all, may be used. Clients who are having problems fulfilling tasks may be given less to do—perhaps therapists return to an earlier program week or stop the program altogether for awhile. Those finding food-planning impossible (they travel much, live in a dormitory) may calorie plan.

Appendix 3:
Recommended Dietary
Allowances*

Food and Nutrition Board, National Academy of Sciences-National Research Council Recommended Daily Dietary Allowances,[a] Revised 1980

Designed for the maintenance of good nutrition of practically all healthy people in the U.S.A.

	Age (years)	Weight (kg)	Weight (lb)	Height (cm)	Height (in)	Protein (g)	Fat-Soluble Vitamins Vitamin A (µg re)[b]	Vitamin D (µg)[c]	Vitamin E (mg α-TE)[d]	Water-Soluble Vitamins Vitamin C (mg)	Thiamin (mg)	Riboflavin (mg)	Niacin (mg NE)[e]	Vitamin B-6 (mg)	Folacin[f] (µg)	Vitamin B-12 (µg)
Infants	0.0–0.5	6	13	60	24	kg×2.2	420	10	3	35	0.3	0.4	6	0.3	30	0.5[g]
	0.5–1.0	9	20	71	28	kg×2.0	400	10	4	35	0.5	0.6	8	0.6	45	1.5
Children	1–3	13	29	90	35	23	400	10	5	45	0.7	0.8	9	0.9	100	2.0
	4–6	20	44	112	44	30	500	10	6	45	0.9	1.0	11	1.3	200	2.5
	7–10	28	62	132	52	34	700	10	7	45	1.2	1.4	16	1.6	300	3.0
Males	11–14	45	99	157	62	45	1000	10	8	50	1.4	1.6	18	1.8	400	3.0
	15–18	66	145	176	69	56	1000	10	10	60	1.4	1.7	18	2.0	400	3.0
	19–22	70	154	177	70	56	1000	7.5	10	60	1.5	1.7	19	2.2	400	3.0
	23–50	70	154	178	70	56	1000	5	10	60	1.4	1.6	18	2.2	400	3.0
	51+	70	154	178	70	56	1000	5	10	60	1.2	1.4	16	2.2	400	3.0
Females	11–14	46	101	157	62	46	800	10	8	50	1.1	1.3	15	1.8	400	3.0
	15–18	55	120	163	64	46	800	10	8	60	1.1	1.3	14	2.0	400	3.0
	19–22	55	120	163	64	44	800	7.5	8	60	1.1	1.3	14	2.0	400	3.0
	23–50	55	120	163	64	44	800	5	8	60	1.0	1.2	13	2.0	400	3.0
	51+	55	120	163	64	44	800	5	8	60	1.0	1.2	13	2.0	400	3.0
Pregnant						+30	+200	+5	+2	+20	+0.4	+0.3	+2	+0.6	+400	+1.0
Lactating						+20	+400	+5	+3	+40	+0.5	+0.5	+5	+0.5	+100	+1.0

	Age (years)	Weight (kg)	Weight (lb)	Height (cm)	Height (in)	Protein (g)	Calcium (mg)	Phosphorus (mg)	Magnesium (mg)	Iron (mg)	Zinc (mg)	Iodine (µg)
Infants	0.0–0.5	6	13	60	24	kg × 2.2	360	240	50	10	3	40
	0.5–1.0	9	20	71	28	kg × 2.0	540	360	70	15	5	50
Children	1–3	13	29	90	35	23	800	800	150	15	10	70
	4–6	20	44	112	44	30	800	800	200	10	10	90
	7–10	28	62	132	52	34	800	800	250	10	10	120
Males	11–14	45	99	157	62	45	1200	1200	350	18	15	150
	15–18	66	145	176	69	56	1200	1200	400	18	15	150
	19–22	70	154	177	70	56	800	800	350	10	15	150
	23–50	70	154	178	70	56	800	800	350	10	15	150
	51+	70	154	178	70	56	800	800	350	10	15	150
Females	11–14	46	101	157	62	46	1200	1200	300	18	15	150
	15–18	55	120	163	64	46	1200	1200	300	18	15	150
	19–22	55	120	163	64	44	800	800	300	18	15	150
	23–50	55	120	163	64	44	800	800	300	18	15	150
	51+	55	120	163	64	44	800	800	300	10	15	150
Pregnant						+30	+400	+400	+150	h	+5	+25
Lactating						+20	+400	+400	+150	h	+10	+50

[a]The allowances are intended to provide for individual variations among most normal persons as they live in the United States under usual environmental stresses. Diets should be based on a variety of common foods in order to provide other nutrients for which human requirements have been less well defined.

[b]Retinol equivalents. 1 retinol equivalent = 1 µg retinol or 6 µg β carotene.

[c]As cholecalciferol. 10 µg cholecalciferol = 400 IU of vitamin D.

[d]α-tocopherol equivalents. 1 mg d-α tocopherol = 1-α-TE.

[e]1 NE (niacin equivalent) is equal to 1 mg of niacin or 60 mg of dietary tryptophan.

[f]The folacin allowances refer to dietary sources as determined by *Lactobacillus casei* assay after treatment with enzymes (conjugases) to make polyglutamyl forms of the vitamin available to the test organism.

[g]The recommended dietary allowance for vitamin B-12 in infants is based on average concentration of the vitamin in human milk. The allowances after weaning are based on energy intake (as recommended by the American Academy of Pediatrics) and consideration of other factors, such as intestinal absorption.

[h]The increased requirement during pregnancy cannot be met by the iron content of habitual American diets nor by the existing iron stores of many women; therefore the use of 30–60 mg of supplemental iron is recommended. Iron needs during lactation are not substantially different from those of nonpregnant women, but continued supplementation of the mother for 2–3 months after parturition is advisable in order to replenish stores depleted by pregnancy.

*Source of data: Committee on Dietary Allowances, Food and Nutrition Board, National Academy of Sciences, 1980.

Appendix 4:
Manitoba Obesity
Clinic Interview*

Name _____

Age _____ Yr _____ Months _____ Birthdate _____ 19 _____

Height _____ in _____ cm   Height and weight of all family

Weight _____ lb _____ kg   members _____

_____

Menstrual cycle data: Time of month _____

Education _____ Do you gain weight before it?

Occupation _____ How much _____

Parents: Education: Mother _____ Father _____

　　　　 Occupation: Mother _____ Father _____

Raised by (1) both parents (2) Mother (3) Father (4) other _____

Residence (1) with family (2) with spouse (3) alone (4) with
　　　　friends—how many? _____ (5) in room and board situation (6) in
　　　　university residence (7) other _____

If married with family, how many children? _____

Past and Present

Age of obesity onset (when did it first become a problem?)

Are any family members or close relatives overweight? (1) Yes (2) No

If yes, which ones, for how long, when did it become a problem with
　　　　them, and how much overweight?

Are you currently in a period of weight gain or weight loss or are you
　　　　maintaining a constant weight?

_____

*See also the Stanford Eating Disorders Questionnaire (Agras, 1987).

110

What has been your past history of weight loss and regain?
What has been your history of dieting attempts and practices and does
    this relate to your history of weight loss and gain?
Have any negative effects (e.g., feeling bad, etc.) accompanied previous
    dieting attempts?
Are you currently taking any medications? What are they? Are they
    physician or self-prescribed?
Past medical history—any illness, operations, accompanying medica-
    tions, and were there any weight changes accompanying these?
Do you currently have arthritis, heart disease, diabetes, gall bladder
    disease or any other medical conditions?

Eating Practices—General

Do you snack a lot? (What constitutes these snacks?)
Do you eat junk food (soft drinks, choc. bars, etc.), when, and how
    much?
Typically:

Do you eat breakfast? (1) Yes (when, where, what) (2) No
Do you eat lunch?   (1) Yes (when, where, what) (2) No
Do you eat dinner?   (1) Yes (when, where, what) (2) No
Who does the shopping for food?
Who prepares the meals?
Is there anyone in the home who requires special meals (e.g., a diabetic)
    and does this affect the others' diets?
Are meals taken alone or with family or friends?
    Breakfast _____
    Lunch _____
    Dinner _____
    Snacks _____
Are mealtimes pleasant? Which are the most pleasant and why?
How much out-of-home eating occurs?
    when _____
    why_____
    what _____
    with whom _____
How much alcoholic beverage consumption occurs, what kinds, and
    with whom?
When shopping, at a movie, or watching TV do you eat anything?
What?

Exercise Practices

Do you have any opportunities for regular planned exercise?
Do you purposely set times aside to exercise?
Do you do special exercises—where, when, with whom?
Do you participate in any sports—how often, where, and with whom?
Do you like exercising?
If you don't exercise, why not?
How much walking do you do?
Do you use elevators or stairs?
Is your residence on ground level? If not how many stairs must you climb? Is there an elevator and do you use it?
Are there stairs in your residence? Do you use them? How many times a day?
Are there many labor-saving devices in your home? Do you use them and what are they?
How much TV do you watch?
Do you walk to post a letter, go to the store, or do you drive or take a bus?
Do you walk to post a letter, go to the store, or do you drive or take a bus? How far is it?
Do you prefer going for a car ride or for a walk in your spare time?
Do you bicycle? If yes, how much, when, and with whom?
Are there any situations in which you exercise more than usual?
Are there any situations in which you exercise less than usual?
What has your past pattern of exercise and sports participation been?

Nutrition

What constitutes good nutrition to you?
Do you think you have adequate nutrition?
Do you take vitamin and mineral supplements?

Problem Areas

Do you think you're overweight? If so, why?
Detail situations which are particularly problematic.

Appendix 5:
Physician Permission Form

Name of Client _____ Date _____

    The person named above wishes to participate in the Manitoba Obesity Clinic program. The regimen he or she will undergo includes both dieting and exercising and will be conducted at the University of Manitoba. Please inform us if there is any medical reason that the above-named person should not undergo this weight loss program or if there are any medical concerns you have about what we intend to do.

    According to my knowledge, there is no medical reason or reasons that would prevent the person named from participating.

                  Physician's Signature _____
                  Date _____

For information about the program please call:

Therapist's Name _____ Phone _____

Appendix 6:
Calorie Expenditure Values*

EXERCISE (APPROXIMATE)	NUMBER OF CALORIES EXPENDED PER MINUTE BY 150-LB PERSON
Badminton	5.8
Baseball	4.7
Basketball	
Moderate Play	7
Fast Play	8.5
Biking	
Leisurely (5 mph)	5
Fast (13 mph)	10.8
Canoeing	
Slow (2.5 mph)	3
Faster (4 mph)	7
Dancing	
Moderate	4
Fast	6
Football	8.4
Golf	
Foursome	4.1
Twosome	5.5
Handball (vigorous)	10
Jogging (see running below)	
Ping Pong	3.9
Racquetball	10
Rope Jumping	12.5
Running	
slow (12 min/mile)	10
faster (8 min/mile)	15
(6 min/mile)	20
Skating	
ice-skating	11.5
roller-skating	11.5
Skiing	
Cross Country	
Leisurely	9
Moderately	11.8
Fast Pace (8 mph)	17
Downhill	8–10
Water	7.8
Snowshoeing (2.5 mph)	9
Soccer	9
Squash	10
Swimming (leisurely)	6
Tennis	
Recreational	7
Fast	9.8
Walking	
Stroll (2 mph) level	3.5
Fair Clip (3 mph+)	5
Uphill on 5% grade	7.5 (increase with steepness)
Hiking heavy pack level plane (3 mph+)	6.8
Hiking uphill	9.8
Walking on snow (Reasonably hard at 3 mph+)	10

*Source of Data: Fitness Finders, 1969; Larsen & Michelman, 1973; Sharkey, 1974.

Appendix 7:
Algorithm for
Adjusting Calories

1. Activity _____

2. Rate of expenditure per min (at 150 lb) _____

3. Planned min of activity _____

4. Expended calories at 150 lb (step 2 times step 3) _____

5. 10% of step 4 _____

6. Client's current weight _____

7. Fifteen-pound units (e.g., 1, 2, 3) over or under 150 lbs the client is currently _____

8. Adjustment of calories (step 5 times step 7) _____

9. Expenditure of calories after adjusting (Add steps 8 and 4 if client heavier than 150 lbs. Subtract step 8 from step 4 if client lighter than 150 lbs.) _____

Appendix 8:
Violation Themes*

EATING

Theme	Definition
1. Food Friend	Food proffered by another to be hospitable or nice. The problem is being unable to assertively refuse the offering.
2. Food Reward	Food is eaten to celebrate some triumph.
3. Food Available	Easily obtained because it's omnipresent.
4. Food Presence	Easily obtained because not only omnipresent but in full view.
5. Food Conserved	Food is eaten to avoid storing it or throwing it away.
6. Food Tasting	Calories consumed exceed plans because of tasting the food being prepared.
7. Food Craved	A particular food is sought because one has an urge for it.
8. Food Outing	Foods are eaten out of restricted choice.
9. Others Eating	One eats because others are observed doing so.

10. Time Available   Eating occurs to endure an interval of
                                     time, eating while waiting.

11. Food Heroics   Food is eaten as a result of some past
                                     denial of food or as a reward for an
                                     episode of exercise.

ACTIVITY

Theme   Definition

1. Activity Excessive   Too much is demanded.

2. Too Unimportant for   Allowing others to intrude upon times
   Activity   to be active.

3. Activity Visible   Violating plans because of being
                                     reluctant to be seen (in public)
                                     exercising.

4. Too Busy for Activity   Violating plans because minor tasks
                                     arise and create a sense of urgency that
                                     is undeserved. Or, being unable to plan
                                     to be active because one's schedule
                                     appears to be congested.

5. Forgetting About   No alternative activities or places to be
   Rainy Days   active are available to handle situations
                                     where the client *must* put aside the
                                     original plan.

6. Activity Boring   The activity planned becomes dull—
                                     either the activity is boring, the place
                                     where it occurs is boring, or doing the
                                     activity by oneself is dull.

7. Activity-Sparer   Violating plans because of others or
                                     another who eliminates the possibility
                                     for the client to be active or who insists
                                     on the client taking the least strenuous
                                     route.

---

*Other reasons are possible and combinations likely.

References

Abramson, R., Garg, M., Cioffari, A., & Rottman, P. A. (1980). An evaluation of behavioral techniques reinforced with an anorectic drug in a double blind weight loss study. *Journal of Clinical Psychiatry, 41,* 234–237.

Agras, W. S. (1987). *Eating disorders.* New York: Pergamon Press.

Alberti, R. E., & Emmons, M. L. (1970). *Your perfect right: A guide to assertive behavior.* San Luis Obispo, CA: Impact.

Allon, N. (1980). Sociological aspects of overweight youth. In P. J. Collipp (Ed.), *Childhood obesity* (2nd ed.). Littleton, MA: PSG Publishing.

American College of Sports Medicine. (1978). The recommended quantity and quality of exercise for developing and maintaining fitness in healthy adults. *Medicine and Science in Sports, 10,* 7–10.

Ashwell, M., Priest, P., & Bondoux, M. (1975). Adipose tissue cellularity in obese women. In A. Howard (Ed.), *Recent advances in obesity research: I.* London: Newman Publishing.

Auto-Nutritionist. (1987). Silverton, OR: N2-squared computing.

Baecke, J. A., van Staveren, W. A., & Buremia, J. (1983). Food consumption, habitual physical activity, and body fatness in young Dutch adults. *American Journal of Clinical Nutrition, 37,* 278–286.

Barlow, D. H., Hayes, S. C., & Nelson, R. D. (1984). *The scientist practitioner.* New York: Pergamon Press.

Bellack, A. S. (1975). Behavior therapy for weight reduction. *Addictive Behaviors, 1,* 73–82.

Bellack, A. S., & Rozensky, R. H. (1975). The selection of dependent variables for weight reduction studies. *Journal of Behavior Therapy and Experimental Psychiatry, 6,* 83–84.

Bennett, G. A., & Jones, S. E. (1986). Dropping out of treatment for obesity. *Journal of Psychosomatic Research, 30,* 567–573.

Bernard, J. L. (1968). Rapid treatment of gross obesity by operant techniques. *Psychological Reports, 23,* 663–666.

Bigelow, G. E., Griffiths, R. R., Liebson, I., & Kalizak, J. (1980). Double-blind evaluation of reinforcing and anorectic actions of weight control medications. *Archives of General Psychiatry, 37,* 1118–1123.

Bistrian, B. R., & Sherman, M. (1978). Results of the treatment of obesity with a protein-sparing modified fast. *International Journal of Obesity, 2,* 143–148.

Bjorntorp, P. (1985). Obesity and risk of cardiovascular disease. *Acta Medica Scandinavica, 218,* 145–147.

Bjorntorp, P., Carlgren, G., Isaksson, B., Krotiewski, M., Larsson, B., & Sjostrom, L. (1975). Effect of energy reduced dietary regimen in relation to adipose tissue cellularity in obese women. *American Journal of Clinical Nutrition, 28,* 445–452.

Black, D. R., & Lantz, C. E. (1984). Spouse involvement and a possible long-term follow-up trap in weight loss. *Behaviour Research and Therapy, 22,* 557–562.

Blackburn, G. L., & Pavlou, K. (1984). Fad reducing diets: Separating fads from facts. *Contemporary Nutrition, 8,* 349–351.

Booth, D. A. (1980). Acquired behavior controlling energy intake and output. In A. J. Stunkard (Ed.), *Obesity.* Philadelphia: W. B. Saunders.

Bowerman, W. J., Harris, W. E., & Shea, J. M. (1978). *Jogging.* New York: Grosset and Dunlap.

Bray, G. A. (1976). *The obese patient.* Toronto: W. B. Saunders Company.

Bray, G. A. (1985). Obesity: Definition, diagnosis, and disadvantages. *The Medical Journal of Australia, 142,* special supplement, 52–58.

Brownell, K. D. (1982). Obesity: Understanding and treating a serious, prevalent, and refractory disorder. *Journal of Consulting and Clinical Psychology, 50,* 820–840.

Brownell, K. D. (1987). *The learn program for weight control.* Philadelphia, PA: Author.

Brownell, K. D., & Foreyt, J. P. (1985). Obesity. In D. Barlow (Ed.), *Clinical Handbook of Psychological Disorders.* New York: Guilford.

Brownell, K. D., Heckerman, C. L., Westlake, R. J., Hayes, S. C., & Monti, P. M. (1978). The effect of couples training and partner cooperativeness in the behavioral treatment of obesity. *Behaviour Research and Therapy, 16,* 323–333.

Brownell, K. D., & Jeffery, R. W. (1987). Improving long-term weight loss: Pushing the limits of treatment. *Behavior Therapy, 18,* 353–374.

Brownell, K. D., & Stunkard, A. J. (1981a). Couples training, pharmacotherapy, and behavior therapy in the treatment of obesity. *Archives of General Psychiatry, 38,* 1224–1229.

Brownell, K. D., & Stunkard, A. J. (1981b). Differential changes in plasma high-density lipoprotein-cholesterol levels of obese men and women during weight reduction. *Archives of Internal Medicine, 141,* 1142–1146.

Brownell, K. D., & Stunkard, A. J. (1980). Physical activity in the development and control of obesity. In A. J. Stunkard (Ed.), *Obesity.* Philadelphia: W. B. Saunders.

Brozek, J., & Keys, A. (1951). The evaluation of leanness–fatness in man: Norms and inter-relationships. *British Journal of Nutrition, 5,* 194–206.

Cahnman, W. J. (1968). The stigma of obesity. *Sociological Quarterly, 9,* 283–299.

Carroll, C., Miller, D., & Nash, J. C. (1976). *Health: The science of human adaptation.* Dubuque, IA: Wm. C. Brown.

Cautela, J. R. (1977). *Behavior analysis forms for clinical intervention.* Champaign, IL: Research Press.

Committee on Dietary Allowances (1980). *Recommended dietary allowances* (9th ed.). Washington, DC: National Research Council, National Academy of Sciences.

Craighead, L. W. (1984). Sequencing of behavior therapy and pharmacotherapy for obesity. *Journal of Consulting and Clinical Psychology, 52,* 190–199.

Craighead, L. W., Stunkard, A. J., & O'Brien, R. (1981). Behavior therapy and pharmacotherapy of obesity. *Archives of General Psychiatry, 38,* 763–768.

Davis, J. (1980). *Garfield at large: His first book.* New York: Ballantine Books.

DeJong, W. (1980). The stigma of obesity: The consequences of naive assumptions concerning the causes of physical deviance. *Journal of Health and Social Behavior, 21,* 75–87.

Deutsch, R. M. (1976). *Realities of nutrition.* Palo Alto, CA: Bull Publishing.

Dietz, W. H., Gortmaker, S. L., Sobol, A. M., & Wehler, C. A. (1985). Trends in the prevalence of childhood and adolescent obesity in the United States. *Pediatric Research, 19,* 527 (abstract).

Donahoe, C. P., Lin, D. A., Kirschenbaum, D. S., & Keesey, R. E. (1984). Metabolic consequences of dieting and exercise in the treatment of obesity. *Journal of Consulting and Clinical Psychology, 52,* 827–836.

Donahoe, R. P., Abbott, R. D., Bloom, E., Reed, D. M., & Yano, K. (1987, April 11). Central obesity and coronary heart disease in man. *Lancet, 1,* 821.

Dressendorfer, R. (1975). Lean body mass increase with exercise. *Obesity and Bariatric Medicine, 4,* 188–190.

Dubbert, P. M., & Wilson, G. T. (1984). Goal setting and spouse involvement in the treatment of obesity. *Behaviour Research and Therapy, 22,* 227–242.

Durnin, J. V., & Womersley, J. (1974). Body fat assessed from total body density and its estimation from skinfold thickness: Measurements on 481 men and women aged 16–72 years. *British Journal of Nutrition, 32,* 77–97.

Edelman, B. (1982). Developmental differences in the conceptualization of obesity. *Journal of the American Dietetic Association, 80,* 122–126.

Edwards, D. W. W., Hammond, W. H., Healy, M. L. R., Tanner, T. M., & Whitehouse, R. H. (1955). Design and accuracy of calipers for measuring subcutaneous tissue thickness. *British Journal of Nutrition, 9,* 133–143.

Epstein, L. H., Masek, B. J., & Marshall, W. R. (1978). A nutritionally based school program for control of eating in obese children. *Behavior Therapy, 9,* 766–778.

Epstein, L. H., Wing, R. R., & Valoski, A. (1985). Childhood obesity. *Pediatric Clinics of North America, 32,* 363–379.

Eufemia, R. L., & Wesoloski, M. D. (1985). Attrition in behavioral studies of obesity: A meta-analytic review. *The Behavior Therapist, 8,* 115–116.

Feinstein, A. R. (1959). The measurement of success in weight reduction: An analysis of methods and a new index. *Journal of Chronic Diseases, 10,* 439–456.

Ferster, C. B., Nurnberger, I. I., & Levitt, E. B. (1962). The control of eating. *Journal of Mathetics, 1,* 87–109.

Fitness Finders. (1969). *A unique approach to personal fitness.* Pennsylvania, PA: Author.

Fitzgerald, F. I. (1985). Space-age snake oil: Obesity and consumer fraud. *Postgraduate Medicine, 78,* 231–240.

Follick, M. J., Abrams, D. B., Smith, T. W., Henderson, O., & Herbert, P. N. (1984). Contrasting short- and long-term effects of weight loss on lipoprotein levels. *Archives of Internal Medicine, 144,* 1571–1574.

Food and Agriculture Organization (FAO) (1977). *Dietary fats and oils in human nutrition.* Report of FAO Expert Committee. FAO Food and Nutrition Paper No. 3. Rome, Italy: Author.

Forbes, G. B. (1962). Methods for determining composition of the human body. *Pediatrics, 29,* 477–494.

Forman, M. R., Trowbridge, F. L., Gentry, E. M., Marks, J. S., & Hogelin, G. C. (1986). Overweight adults in the United States: The behavioral risk factor surveys. *The American Journal of Clinical Nutrition, 44,* 410–416.

Garn, S. M. (1985). Continuities and changes in fatness from infancy through adulthood. *Current Problems in Pediatrics, 15,* 5–47.

Garn, S. M., & Clark, D. C. (1975). Nutrition, growth, development, and maturation: Findings from the ten-state nutrition survey of 1968–1970. *Pediatrics, 56,* 306–319.

Garn, S. M., Clark, D. C., & Guire, K. E. (1975). Growth, body composition, and development of obese and lean children. In M. Winick (Ed.), *Childhood obesity.* New York: John Wiley & Sons.

Garn, S. M., Hopkins, P. J., & Ryan, A. S. (1981). Differential fatness gain of low income boys and girls. *The American Journal of Clinical Nutrition, 34,* 1465–1468.

Garn, S. M., Sullivan, T. V., & Hawthorne, V. M. (1987, June 20). Does "central" obesity predict coronary artery disease? *The Lancet, 1,* 1438–1439.

Garrison, R. J., Wilson, P. J., Castelli, W. P., Fenleib, M., Kannel, W. B., & McNamara, P. M.

(1980). Obesity and lipoprotein cholesterol in the Framingham Offspring Study. *Metabolism, 29,* 1053–1060.

Garrow, J. S. (1974). *Energy balance and obesity in man.* New York: Elsevier.

Garrow, J. S. (1978a). *Energy balance and obesity in man* (2nd ed.) Amsterdam: Elsevier.

Garrow, J. S. (1978b). The regulation of energy expenditure in man. In G. A. Bray (Ed.), *Recent advances in obesity research: II.* London: Newman Publishing.

Goldblatt, P. B., Moore, M. E., & Stunkard, A. J. (1965). Social factors in obesity. *Journal of the American Medical Association, 192,* 1039–1044.

Goldman, R. F., & Buskirk, E. R. (1959). Body volume measurement by underwater weighing: Description of a method. In J. Brozek & A. Heneschel (Eds.), *Techniques for measuring body composition.* Washington, DC: National Academy of Sciences.

Grimes, W. B., & Franzini, L. R. (1977). Skinfold measurement techniques for estimating percentage of body fat. *Journal of Behavior Therapy and Experimental Psychiatry, 8,* 65–69.

Gurr, M. I., & Kirtland, J. (1978). Adipose tissue cellularity—a review: I. Techniques for studying cellularity. *International Journal of Obesity, 2,* 401–427.

Hagen, R. L., Foreyt, J. P., & Durham, T. W. (1976). The dropout problem: Reducing attrition in obesity research. *Behavior Therapy, 7,* 463–471.

Hirsch, J. (1975). Cell number and size as a determinant of subsequent obesity. In M. Winnick (Ed.), *Childhood obesity.* New York: John Wiley & Sons.

Jamieson, M. G. (1987). Obesity and hypertensive cardiovascular disease. *The Journal of the American Medical Association, 258,* 323.

Jeffery, R. W. (1987). Behavioral treatment of obesity. *Annals of Behavioral Medicine, 9,* 20–23.

Jeffery, R. W., Bjornson-Benson, W. M., Rosenthal, B. S., Lindquist, R. A., Kurth, C. L., & Johnson, S. I. (1984). Calorie requirements in weight loss: An estimate based on self-reported food intake in middle-aged men. *Addictive Behaviors, 9,* 231–233.

Jeffery, R. W., Gerber, W. M., Rosenthal, B. S., & Lindquist, R. A. (1983). Monetary contracts in weight control: Effectiveness of group and individual contracts of varying size. *Journal of Consulting and Clinical Psychology, 51,* 242–248.

Jeffery, R. W., Thompson, P. D., & Wing, R. R. (1978). Effects on weight reduction of strong monetary contracts for calorie restriction or weight loss. *Behaviour Research and Therapy, 16,* 363–369.

Jeffery, R. W., Wing, R. R., & Stunkard, A. J. (1978). Behavioral treatment of obesity: The state of the art. *Behavior Therapy, 9,* 189–199.

Jeffrey, D. B., & Katz, R. C. (1977). *Take it off and keep it off: A behavioral program for weight loss and healthy living.* Englewood Cliffs, NJ: Prentice-Hall.

Johnson, R. E., Mastropaolo, J. A., & Wharton, M. A. (1972). Exercise, dietary intake, and body composition. *Journal of the American Dietetic Association, 61,* 399–403.

Jones, P. R. M., Hunt, M. J., Brown, T. P., & Norgan, N. G. (1986). Waist–hip circumference ratio and its relation to age and overweight in British men. *Human Nutrition: Clinical Nutrition, 40C,* 239–247.

Jordan, H. A. (1973). In defense of body weight. *Journal of the American Dietetic Association, 62,* 17–21.

Jordan, H. A., Levitz, L. S., & Kimbrell, G. M. (1976). In S. Gelman (Ed.), *Eating is okay.* New York: Rawson Associates Publishers, Inc.

Kanfer, F. H. (1970). Self-monitoring: Methodological limitations and clinical applications. *Journal of Consulting and Clinical Psychology, 35,* 148–152.

Kanfer, F. H. (1977). The many faces of self-control, or behavior modification changes its focus. In R. B. Stuart (Ed.), *Behavioral self-management: Strategies, techniques and outcomes.* New York: Brunner/Mazel.

Keesey, R. E. (1980). A set-point analysis of the regulation of body weight. In A. J. Stunkard (Ed.), *Obesity*. Philadelphia, PA: W. B. Saunders Company.

Keesey, R. E., & Corbett, S. W. (1984). Metabolic defense of the body weight set-point. In A. J. Stunkard & E. Stellar (Eds.), *Eating and its disorders*. New York: Raven Press.

Keys, S., Brozek, J., Henschel, F., Mickelson, O., & Taylor, H. L. (1950). *The biology of human starvation* (Vols. 1 & 2). Minneapolis, MN: University of Minnesota Press.

Kiesler, D. J. (1966). Some myths of psychotherapy research and the search for a paradigm. *Psychological Bulletin, 65*, 110–136.

Knittle, J. L. (1975). Basic concepts in the control of childhood obesity. In M. Winick (Ed.), *Childhood obesity*. New York: John Wiley & Sons.

Konoshi, F. (1973). *Exercise equivalent of foods*. Carbondale, IL: Southern Illinois University Press.

Kraus, B. (1979). *Calories and carbohydrates*. New York: Grosset and Dunlap.

Lansky, D., & Brownell, K. D. (1982). Estimates of food quantity and calories: Errors in self-report among obese patients. *American Journal of Clinical Nutrition, 35*, 727–732.

Larsen, L., & Michelman, H. (1973). *International guide to fitness and health*. New York: Crown.

LeBow, M. D. (1977). Can lighter become thinner? *Addictive Behaviors, 2*, 87–93.

LeBow, M. D. (1981). *Weight control: The behavioral strategies*. Chichester and New York: John Wiley & Sons.

LeBow, M. D. (1984). *Child obesity*. New York: Springer.

LeBow, M. D. (1986). Child obesity: Dangers. *Canadian Psychology/Psychologie Canadienne, 27*, 275–285.

LeBow, M. D. (in press). *The thin plan*. Champaign, IL: Human Kinetics.

LeBow, M. D., & Lombardi, A. (1986). *Attitudes, perceptions, and practices of Canadian children towards obesity*. Paper presented at the meeting of the Western Psychological Association, Anaheim, California.

Lerner, R. M., & Korn, S. J. (1972). The development of body-build stereotypes in males. *Child Development, 43*, 908–920.

Lindner, P. G. (1974). Exercising the overweight: An exercise in futility? In W. L. Asher (Ed.), *Treating the obese*. Englewood, CL: Medicom Press.

Lindner, P. G., & Blackburn, G. L. (1976). Multidisciplinary approach to obesity utilizing fasting modified by protein-sparing therapy. *Obesity and Bariatric Medicine, 5*, 198–216.

Lloyd, J. K., & Wolff, O. H. (1980). Overnutrition and obesity. In F. Falkner (Ed.), *Presentation in childhood of health problems in adult life*. Geneva: World Health Organization.

Louderback, L. (1970). *Fat power: Whatever you weigh is right*. New York: Hawthorn Books.

Mahoney, M. J. (1975). Fat fiction. *Behavior Therapy, 6*, 416–418.

Mahoney, M. J., & Jeffrey, D. B. (1974). A manual of self-control procedures for the overweight. *JSAS Catalog of Selected Documents in Psychology, 4*, 129.

Mahoney, M. J., & Mahoney, K. (1976). *Permanent weight control*. New York: Norton & Company.

Mann, R. A. (1972). The behavior-therapeutic use of contingency contracting to control an adult behavior problem: Weight control. *Journal of Applied Behavior Analysis, 5*, 99–109.

Manson, J. E., Stampfer, M. J., Hennekens, C. H., & Willett, W. C. (1987). Body weight and longevity: A reassessment. *Journal of the American Medical Association, 257*, 353–361.

Marlatt, G. A., & Gordon, J. R. (1980). Determinants of relapse: Implication for the maintenance of behavior change. In P. O. Davidson & S. M. Davidson (Eds.), *Behavioral medicine: Changing health lifestyles*. New York: Brunner/Mazel.

Marlatt, G. A., & Gordon, J. (1984). *Relapse prevention: A self control strategy for the maintenance of behavior change*. New York: Guilford Press.

Mayer, J. (1968). *Overweight: Causes, cost and control*. Englewood Cliffs, NJ: Prentice-Hall.

Mayer, J., Roy, P., & Mitra, K. P. (1956). Relation between calorie intake, body weight and physical work: Studies in an industrial male population in West Bengal. *American Journal of Clinical Nutrition, 4*, 169–175.

McFall, R. M. (1977). Parameters of self-monitoring. In R. B. Stuart (Ed.), *Behavioral self-management: Strategies, techniques and outcome*. New York: Brunner/Mazel.

McReynolds, W. T., Lutz, R. N., Paulsen, B. K., & Kohrs, M. B. (1975). Treatment manual for the food management (stimulus control) treatment. *JSAS Catalog of Selected Documents in Psychology, 5*, 286.

Meichenbaum, D. (1985). *Stress inoculation training*. New York: Pergamon Press.

Messerli, F. H. (1984). Obesity in hypertension: How innocent a bystander? *The American Journal of Medicine, 77*, 1077–1082.

Metropolitan Life Insurance Tables for Women and Men (1983). New York: Metropolitan Life Insurance Company.

Moody, D. L., Kollias, J., & Buskirk, E. R. (1968). The effect of a moderate exercise program on body weight and skinfold thickness in overweight college women. *Medicine and Science in Sports, 1*, 75–80.

Moore, C. H., & Crum, B. C. (1969). Weight reduction in a chronic schizophrenic by means of operant conditioning procedures: A case study. *Behaviour Research and Therapy, 7*, 129–131.

Moore, M. E., Stunkard, A. J., & Srole, L. (1962). Obesity, social class and mental illness. *Journal of the American Medical Association, 181*, 962–966.

Murphy, J. K., Williamson, D. A., Buxton, A., Moody, S. C., Absher, N., & Warner, M. (1982). The long-term effects of spouse involvement upon weight loss and maintenance. *Behavior Therapy, 13*, 681–693.

Nasco (1987). *Lifeform*. Modesto, CA: NASCO.

National Center for Health Statistics (1973). *Plan and operation of the National Health and Nutrition Examination Survey, United States 1971–1973*. Health Services and Mental Health Administration: Washington, D.C. DHEW publication no. (HSM) 73-1310 (Vital and Health Statistics, series 1, no. 10a and 10b).

National Center for Health Statistics (1981). *Plan and operation of the National Health and Nutrition Examination Survey, 1976–1980*. Washington, D.C. US Public Health Service DHHS publication no. (PHS) 81-1317 (Vital and Health Statistics Series 1, no. 15).

National Institutes of Health Consensus Development Conference Statement (1985). *Health implications of obesity, vol. 5*. Washington, DC: U.S. Government Printing Office.

Nisbett, R. E. (1972). Hunger, obesity, and the ventromedial hypothalamus. *Psychological Review, 79*, 433–453.

Nisbett, R. E. (1974). Starvation and the behavior of the obese. In G. A. Bray & J. E. Bethune (Eds.), *Treatment and management of obesity*. New York: Harper & Row.

Nutzinger, D. V., Cayiroglu, S., Sachs, G., & Zapotoczky, H. G. (1985). Emotional problems during weight reduction: Advantages of a combined behavior therapy and antidepressive drug therapy for obesity. *Journal of Behavior Therapy and Experimental Psychiatry, 16*, 217–221.

Oscai, L. B. (1973). The role of exercise in weight control. *Exercise Sport and Scientific Review, 1*, 103–123.

Ost, L. G., & Gostetam, K. G. (1976). Behavioral and pharmacological treatments for obesity: An experimental comparison. *Addictive Behaviors, 1*, 331–338.

Palgi, A., Read, J., Greenberg, I., Hoeffer, M. A., Bistrian, B. R., & Blackburn, G. L. (1985). Multidisciplinary treatment of obesity with a protein-sparing modified fast: Results in 668 outpatients. *American Journal of Public Health, 75*, 1190–1194.

Pearce, J. W. (1980). *The role of spouse involvement in the behavioral treatment of obese women*. Unpublished doctoral dissertation, University of Manitoba.

Pearce, J., LeBow, M. D., & Orchard, J. (1981). Role of spouse involvement in the behavioral treatment of overweight women. *Journal of Consulting and Clinical Psychology, 49*, 236–244.

Pennington, J. A. T., & Nichols-Church, H. (1980). *Food values of portions commonly used* (13th ed.). New York: Harper & Row.

Perri, M. G., Shapiro, R. M., Ludwig, W. W., Twentyman, C. T., & McAdoo, W. G. (1984). Maintenance strategies for the treatment of obesity: An evaluation of relapse prevention training and posttreatment contact by mail and telephone. *Journal of Consulting and Clinical Psychology, 52*, 404–413.

Polivy, J., & Herman, C. P. (1985). Dieting and binging: A causal analysis. *American Psychologist, 40*, 193–201.

Powers, P. S. (1980). *Obesity: The regulation of weight*. Baltimore, MD: Williams & Wilkins.

R D A. (1980). *Recommended dietary allowances* (9th ed.). Washington, DC: National Academy of Sciences.

Rhoads, G. G., Gulbrandsen, C. L., & Kagan, A. (1976). Serum lipoproteins and coronary heart disease in a population study of Hawaiian-Japanese men. *New England Journal of Medicine, 294*, 293–298.

Richardson, S. A., Goodman, N., Hastorf, A. H., & Dornbusch, S. M. (1961). Cultural uniformity in reaction to physical disabilities. *American Sociological Review, 26*, 241–247.

Roche, A. F. (1981). The adipocyte-number hypothesis. *Child Development, 52*, 31–43.

Rodin, J., Elias, M., Silberstein, L. R., & Wagner, A. (1988). Combined behavioral and pharmacologic treatment for obesity: Predictors of successful weight maintenance. *Journal of Consulting and Clinical Psychology, 56*, 399–404.

Salans, L. B., Cushman, S. W., & Weismann, R. R. (1973). Studies on human tissue: Adipose cell size and number in nonobese and obese patients. *The Journal of Clinical Investigation, 52*, 929–941.

Seltzer, C. C., & Mayer, J. (1965). A simple criterion of obesity. *Postgraduate Medicine, 38*, A101–A107.

Sharkey, B. J. (1974). *Physiological fitness and weight control*. Missoula, MT: Mountain Press.

Sharkey, B. J. (1984). *Physiology of fitness* (2nd ed.). Champaign, IL: Human Kinetics.

Simopoulos, A. (1986). Obesity and body weight standards. *Annual Review of Public Health, 7*, 481–492.

Sims, E. A. H., & Horton, E. S. (1968). Endocrine and metabolic adaptation to obesity and starvation. *American Journal of Clinical Nutrition, 21*, 1455–1470.

Sjostrom, L. (1980). Fat cells and bodyweight. In A. J. Stunkard (Ed.), *Obesity*. Philadelphia: W. B. Saunders Company.

Sperduto, W. A., & O'Brien, R. M. (1983). Effects of cash deposits on attendance and weight loss in a large-scale clinical program for obesity. *Psychological Reports, 52*, 261–262.

Srole, L., Langer, T. S., Michael, S. T., Opler, M. K., & Rennie, T. A. C. (1962). *Mental health in the metropolis: The midtown Manhattan study*. New York: McGraw-Hill.

Staffieri, J. R. (1967). A study of social stereotype of body image in children. *Journal of Personality and Social Psychology, 7*, 101–104.

Stalonas, P. M., & Kirschenbaum, D. S. (1980, November). *Are changes in eating habits associated with weight loss?* Paper presented at meeting of the Society of Behavioral Medicine, New York.

Stern, J. S. (1984). Is obesity a disease of inactivity? In A. J. Stunkard & E. Stellar (Eds.), *Eating and its disorders*. New York: Raven Press.

Stokes, T. F., & Baer, D. M. (1977). An implicit technology of generalization. *Journal of Applied Behavior Analysis, 10*, 349–367.

Stuart, R. B. (1967). Behavioral control of overeating. *Behaviour Research and Therapy, 5*, 357–365.

Stuart, R. B. (1971). A three dimensional program for the treatment of obesity. *Behaviour Research and Therapy, 9,* 177–186.

Stuart, R. B. (1978a). *Act thin, stay thin.* New York: Norton.

Stuart, R. B. (1978b). Workshop on treating obesity. Presented at the Banff Conference on Behavior Modification (Banff 10), Banff, Alberta.

Stuart, R. B., & Davis, B. (1972). *Slim chance in a fat world: Behavioral control of obesity.* Champaign, IL: Research Press.

Stunkard, A. J. (1984). The current status of treatment of obesity in adults. In A. J. Stunkard & E. Stellar (Eds.), *Eating and its disorders.* New York: Raven Press.

Stunkard, A. J. (1985). Behavioral management of obesity. *The Medical Journal of Australia* (special supplement), *142,* 513–520.

Stunkard, A. J., & Rush, J. (1974). Dieting and depression reexamined: A critical review of reports of untoward responses during weight reduction for obesity. *Annals of Internal Medicine, 81,* 526–533.

The Nutrition Company (1984). *Eyeballing the diet.* Tallahassee, FL: Author.

Thompson, J. K., Jarvie, G. J., Lahey, B. B., & Cureton, K. J. (1982). Exercise and obesity: Etiology, physiology, and intervention. *Psychological Bulletin, 91,* 55–79.

Thompson, P. D., Jeffery, R. W., Wing, R. R., & Wood, P. (1979). Unexpected decrease in plasma high density lipoprotein cholesterol with weight loss. *American Journal of Clinical Nutrition, 32,* 2016–2021.

Van Itallie, T. B. (1985). Health implications of overweight and obesity in the United States. *Annals of Internal Medicine, 103,* 983–988.

Vital and Health Statistics (1983, February). *Obese and overweight adults in the United States.* National Center for Health Statistics, Series II, No. 230.

Wadden, T. A. (1987). Very-low-calorie diet and behavior therapy. *The Behavior Therapist, 10,* 49–50.

Wadden, T. A., & Stunkard, A. J. (1986). Controlled trial of very low calorie diet, behavior therapy and their combination in the treatment of obesity. *Journal of Consulting and Clinical Psychology, 54,* 482–488.

Wadden, T. A., Stunkard, A. J., Brownell, K. D., & Day S. C. (1985). A comparison of two very-low-calorie diets: Protein-sparing-modified-fast versus protein formula–liquid diet. *The American Journal of Clinical Nutrition, 41,* 533–539.

Whittaker, J. K., & Garbarino, J. (1983). *Social support networks: Informal helping in the human services.* New York: Aldine.

Wilson, G. T. (1978). Methodological considerations in treatment outcome research on obesity. *Journal of Consulting and Clinical Psychology, 46,* 687–702.

Wilson, G. T., & Brownell, K. D. (1980). Behavior therapy for obesity: An evaluation of treatment outcome. *Advances in Behaviour Research and Therapy, 3,* 49–86.

Wing, R. R., Epstein, L. H., Marcus, M., & Shapira, B. (1981). Strong monetary contingencies for weight loss during treatment and maintenance. *Behavior Therapy, 12,* 702–710.

Wooley, S. C., & Wooley, O. W. (1984). Should obesity be treated at all? In A. J. Stunkard & E. Stellar (Eds.), *Eating and its disorders.* New York: Raven Press.

Zegman, M. (1984). Errors in food recording and calorie estimation: Clinical and theoretical implications for obesity. *Addictive Behaviors, 9,* 347–350.

Zegman, M., & Baker, B. (1983). The influence of proximal vs. distal goals on adherence to prescribed calories. *Addictive Behaviors, 8,* 319–322.

Zuti, W. B. (1972). *Effects of diet and exercise on body composition of adult women during weight reduction.* Unpublished doctoral dissertation, Kent State University.

Zuti, W. B., & Golding, L. A. (1973). Effect of diet and exercise on body composition of adult women during weight reduction. *Medicine and Science in Sports, 5,* 62.

Author Index

Subject Index

About the Author

Michael D. LeBow (PhD, University of Utah) is Professor of Psychology at the University of Manitoba, a clinical psychologist in private practice, and director of the Manitoba Obesity Clinic. He is also on staff at the university's Psychological Service Centre. Dr. LeBow has published seven other books and dozens of scientific articles based on his research and clinical work. His scholarly interests include the study of obesity and society's reactions to it. Dr. LeBow's work with those having weight management problems began while on the faculty of the Department of Psychiatry at Dartmouth Medical School; but his concern with the topic of obesity started years earlier, being rooted in his own experiences as an overweight child and teenager. Dr. LeBow lives in Winnipeg with his wife, Barbara, and two sons, Bill and Matt.

Psychology Practitioner Guidebooks

Editors
Arnold P. Goldstein, Syracuse University
Leonard Krasner, Stanford University & SUNY at Stony Brook
Sol L. Garfield, Washington University in St. Louis

William L. Golden, E. Thomas Dowd & Fred Friedberg—
HYPNOTHERAPY: A Modern Approach

Patricia Lacks—BEHAVIORAL TREATMENT FOR PERSISTENT
INSOMNIA

Arnold P. Goldstein & Harold Keller—AGGRESSIVE BEHAVIOR:
Assessment and Intervention

C. Eugene Walker, Barbara L. Bonner & Keith L. Kaufman—
THE PHYSICALLY AND SEXUALLY ABUSED CHILD: Evaluation
and Treatment

Robert E. Becker, Richard G. Heimberg & Alan S. Bellack—SOCIAL
SKILLS TRAINING TREATMENT FOR DEPRESSION

Richard F. Dangel & Richard A. Polster—TEACHING CHILD
MANAGEMENT SKILLS

Albert Ellis, John F. McInerney, Raymond DiGiuseppe & Raymond
Yeager—RATIONAL-EMOTIVE THERAPY WITH ALCOHOLICS
AND SUBSTANCE ABUSERS

Johnny L. Matson & Thomas H. Ollendick—ENHANCING CHILDREN'S
SOCIAL SKILLS: Assessment and Training

Edward B. Blanchard, John E. Martin & Patricia M. Dubbert—NON-DRUG
TREATMENTS FOR ESSENTIAL HYPERTENSION

Samuel M. Turner & Deborah C. Beidel—TREATING OBSESSIVE-
COMPULSIVE DISORDER

Alice W. Pope, Susan M. McHale & W. Edward Craighead—SELF-
ESTEEM ENHANCEMENT WITH CHILDREN AND ADOLESCENTS

Jean E. Rhodes & Leonard A. Jason—PREVENTING SUBSTANCE
ABUSE AMONG CHILDREN AND ADOLESCENTS

Gerald D. Oster, Janice E. Caro, Daniel R. Eagen & Margaret A. Lillo—
ASSESSING ADOLESCENTS

Robin C. Winkler, Dirck W. Brown, Margaret van Keppel & Amy
Blanchard—CLINICAL PRACTICE IN ADOPTION

Roger Poppen—BEHAVIORAL RELAXATION TRAINING AND
ASSESSMENT

Michael D. LeBow—ADULT OBESITY THERAPY